Tibetan Medicine

W9-CID-172

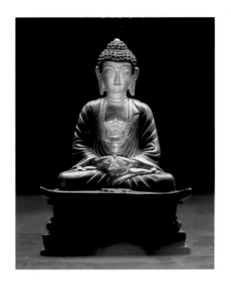

Tibetan Medicine

*A practical and inspirational guide
to diagnosing, treating and
healing the Buddhist Way*

Gerti Samel

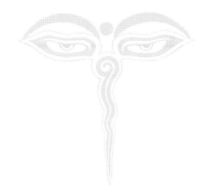

A Little, Brown Book

First published in Great Britain in 2001
by Little, Brown & Company

Copyright © 1998, Mosaik Verlag, München,
part of Verlagsgruppe Random House GmbH
First published as TIBETISCHE MEDIZIN in Germany in 1998 by Mosaik Verlag,
München, part of Verlagsgruppe Random House GmbH

This translation and paperback edition copyright © 2001, Little Brown & Company (UK)

A CIP catalogue record for this book is available from the British Library.

ISBN 0 316 85845 5 (paperback)

Translated by Matthew Barton
Edited, designed and typeset by Grapevine Publishing Services Ltd
Photography: Wolf-Dieter Böttcher, Enno Kapitza, Beatrice Kunzi
Styling: Helge Stussel-Harzer
Printed and bound in Italy by LEGO S.p.a.

Little, Brown & Company (UK)
Brettenham House, Lancaster Place
London WC2E 7EN

Acknowledgments

I would like to thank the following for their help:

Jeanette Häusermann-Cotar of Zurich for her
assistance in describing the Kum-Nye exercises

Matthias Steurich of Freiburg for information and
advice on Kum Nye

Antonia Yeshe Dechen Strub-Tusch of Pfäffikon and
her daughter Dolma Gallmann of Zurich for help with
the physical exercises

Ingrid Samuel for research and assistance with
chapters I and II

Elisabeth McHugh of Küsnacht, Switzerland, for
drawing up the list of plants in the 'Practical
Applications' section of the book

Dr Namgyal Qussar of Dharamsala for medical
information and advice on the constitutional types
and self-treatment

Dr Walburg Maric-Oehler MD of Bad Homburg, and
Dr Pasang Yonten Aryaq for supervision of the
project

Dr Kalsang Shak of Baar, Switzerland, for his advice
on Tibetan teas and constitution types

I am also grateful to the Munich Botanical Garden,
Naturland mail order in Germany and Padma AG in
Switzerland for their assistance.

Picture credits:

H.-D Böttcher: 1, 6-7, 12, 20-21, 24, 30, 49, 50, 53,
54-5, 60, 61, 65, 72, 73, 74, 87, 91, 94, 100, 127,
128-9, 132, 146-7, 148, 150, 151, 152-3; E. Kapitza (for
Cosmopolitan): 9, 10, 15, 17, 26, 29, 33, 35, 43, 46,
51, 52, 59, 67, 98, 131, 134, 138, 141, 143, 144, 145,
149; B. Künzi:104-23; Mosaik/Ziegler:126; Serinfia
Publications: 29, 39, 57

Contents

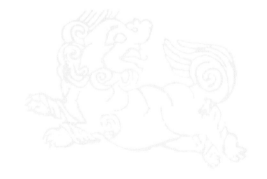

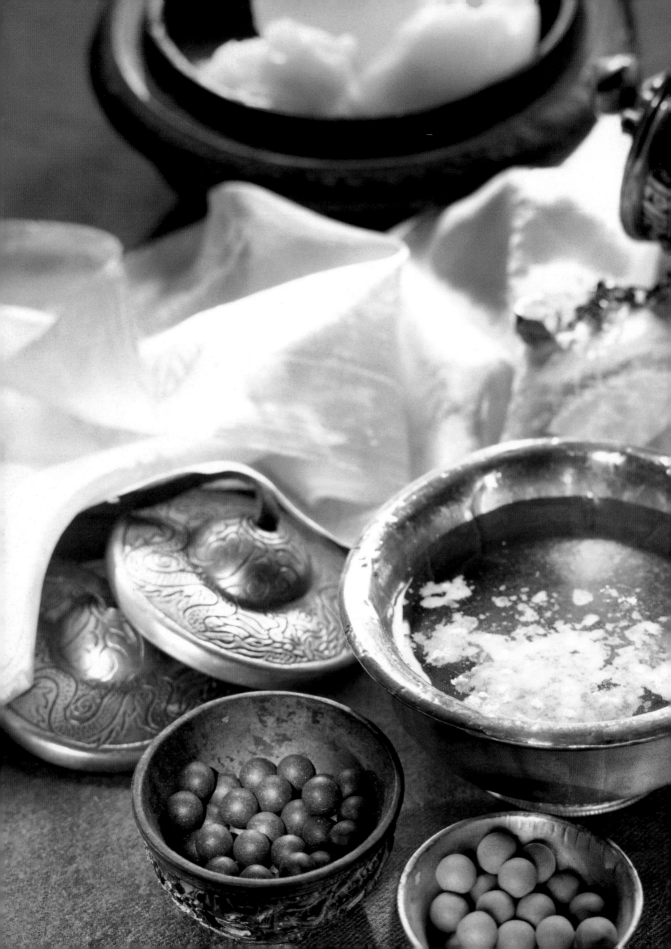

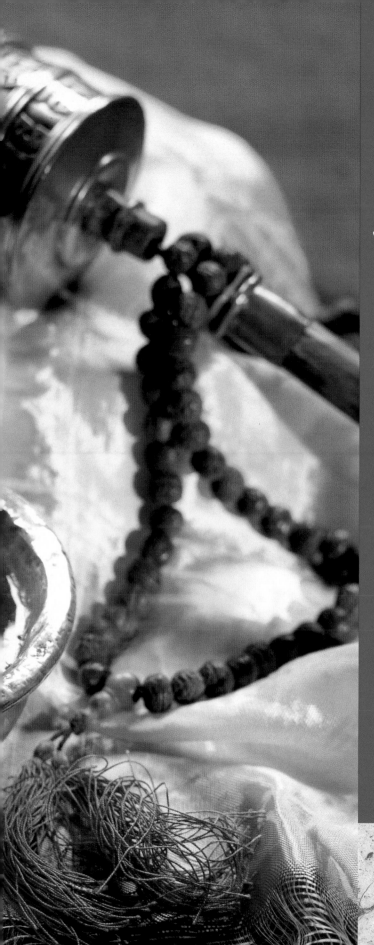

Medicine
from the
Roof of the
World

Chapter 1

THE MYTHOLOGY OF TIBETAN MEDICINE

The land of gold and jewels, source of four great rivers, crowned by the crystal pagoda of the Kailash and adorned with the magic turquoise mirror of Manasarovar.

Ancient Tibetan text

No doubt it has something to do with the land of Tibet itself that the Tibetans' art of healing is so steeped in mythology. Tibet, the great kingdom at the roof of the world, has always been one of the Earth's remotest places. Its magical snow-clad mountains, with peaks of 8,000 metres high, seem to reach close to the gods. Yet thanks to these extreme conditions something unique has been able to evolve, far removed from the rest of the world. Here, just beneath the heavens, a highly developed religious culture emerged over the centuries, whose 'jewel' was a system of medicine that is now providing the West with important new ideas. Based on the Ayurveda, enriched by elements of Chinese medicine and imbued by the whole outlook of Buddhism, Tibetan medicine arose in the highest, most far-flung kingdom of the world. The great masters of Buddhist medical science recorded a 'knowledge of healing' that had been continually refined over the centuries, and preserved it for posterity in written and pictorial form. Tibetan medicine reached a peak in the second half of the 17th century when the 5th Dalai Lama, religious and political leader of the recently reunited realm of Tibet, gave this system of medicine a new form. Since then it has altered very little.

The sufferings of the Tibetan people

A new chapter in Tibet's history began within living memory: in 1950 the Chinese invaded the country and in the Cultural Revolution that followed, Tibetans suffered a holocaust. The Chinese tried to annihilate their entire culture, religion and system of medicine. Tibet is still annexed by China and this political situation has overshadowed Tibetans' lives and destinies ever since. Tibetan medicine has also been affected by the dramatic events that occurred during this period.

In 1949, when the People's Republic of China was proclaimed, the new rulers immediately laid claim to Tibet. The following year the People's Liberation Army invaded, supposedly to free Tibet from the 'poison of imperialism and religion'. Since Tibet was politically isolated and not a member of the United Nations, all appeals to the UN remained ineffectual.

Previous pages – Religion, ritual and healing are closely linked in Tibetan medicine. Shown here are herb pills, cymbals, the traditional white greeting bowl, prayer wheel and rosary. In the centre is the Tibetans' national drink: butter tea with tsampa, *a flour made of roasted barley.*
Opposite – Ancient medical texts are wrapped in silk and brocade and stored in the houses's prayer room.

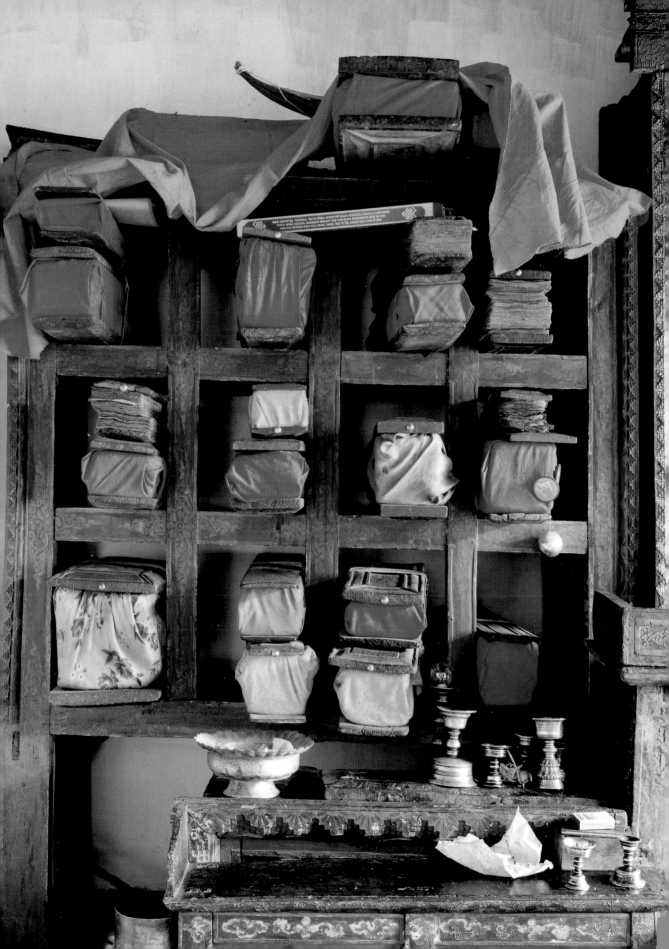

In 1951, a Tibetan delegation was compelled to acknowledge Chinese ascendancy in a 17-point agreement. The 14th Dalai Lama, Tenzin Gyatso (b. 1935), later revoked this, since it had been signed under duress. In response to these events, he was enthroned three years earlier than planned, becoming his people's religious and political leader at the age of 15. Throughout the 1950s, conditions worsened. Despite the Dalai Lama's efforts, the Chinese terror grew so intolerable that in 1959, rebellion broke out in the capital, Lhasa, and was bloodily suppressed.

The Dalai Lama takes flight

When rumours surfaced in March 1959 that the Chinese were planning to abduct the Dalai Lama, many thousands of people flocked to his summer palace, the Norbulinka, to protect him. By the end of that month, before the Chinese opened fire on his palace, the Dalai Lama had fled to northern India. All influential Tibetans remaining in the country were taken prisoner. In the Cultural Revolution that followed, it is estimated that a million Tibetans lost their lives while around

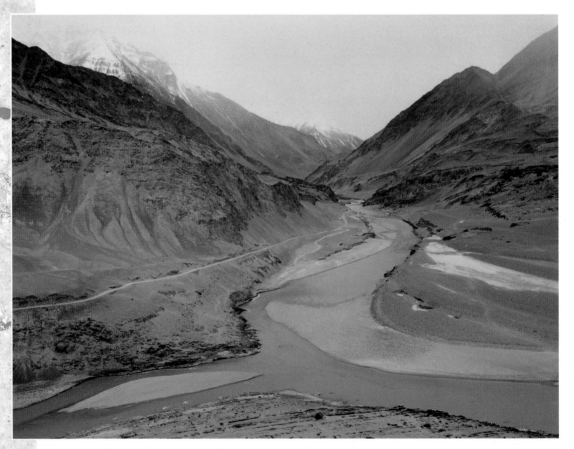

The roof of the world: the snow peaks of Ladakh and the river Indus

80,000 fled to Nepal and India. In the next few years, 6,000 Tibetan monasteries were razed to the ground, and most Tibetan religious culture was destroyed. Since many monastery schools were also centres of medical learning, the Chinese rulers ruthlessly wiped out almost all Tibetan medical knowledge. Tibet's most important school of medicine, Chagpori, on the iron hill of Lhasa, was reduced to dust and ashes. Tibetan doctors of the older generation were taken prisoner, and most of them subsequently died in captivity from the effects of forced labour and torture.

It is only thanks to the foresight of a few, great Tibetan scholars that some of the ancient knowledge was preserved. Doctors used to have to learn the ancient medical texts by heart during their studies, so it was possible to reconstruct them from memory and record them on paper once more.

A new home in Indian exile

The 14th Dalai Lama settled in the northern Indian mountain village of Dharamsala. At the foot of the Indian Himalayas, 1,800 metres above sea level, he founded his government in exile, and many Tibetans found a new home with him. Soon new schools of Tibetan culture, religion and medicine grew up. In 1961, the Dalai Lama founded a new medical school in Dharamsala under the direction of his personal physicians. The Tibetan Medical and Astrological Institute (known to Tibetans as the Men-Tsee-Khang) has become, under his auspices, the most important centre for Tibetan medicine in the world. The Institute functions as a centre for training, research, pharmacology, the production of medicines, astrology and, of course, medical treatment based on Tibetan principles.

In the Tibetan Medical and Astrological Institute, a new generation of doctors learned their profession under the supervision of an older generation of teachers, who had trained in Tibet. They then began to spread Tibetan medical wisdom throughout the Western world. Their goal was supported and sustained by the wave of interest in Buddhism that was sweeping Europe and the USA. The Dalai Lama was aware from the outset of the opportunities offered by a rebirth of Tibetan medicine in exile and has guided developments carefully. Doctors were forced to adapt ancient methods to suit new conditions and open themselves to the world, and thus Tibetan medicine has been pursuing new paths.

How the world views Tibetan methods of healing

Western doctors, therapists, botanists and pharmacists are increasingly interested in Tibetan healing arts. The spiritual and intellectual methods it utilizes have been an integral part of Western psychotherapy and physical therapies for many years now. Many scientists are fascinated by the efficacy of Tibetan medicine and convinced that Tibetan plant-lore can show us new paths to healing.

In the treatment of illnesses for which allopathic medicines (the traditional Western approach) have no answer, there are some interesting new ideas coming from the Himalayas. The German doctor Egbert Asshauer, a great expert on Tibetan medicine, believes that Tibetan healing methods should be used in the West to complement orthodox medical practice – and vice versa. Even Tibetans resort to antibiotics in certain cases. The two medical systems could co-exist and enrich each other. This co-existence is already practised in Dharamsala in a very straightforward way: the Delek hospital, where doctors practise orthodox Western medicine, is a few minutes' walk away from the Tibetan Medical and Astrological Institute, and the doctors of each institute frequently refer patients to each other. Patients with tuberculosis or other acute infections go straight to the Delek hospital, while the Tibetan Medical and Astrological Institute is regarded as better for treating chronic conditions.

Why the methods work

Many Western patients have now experienced the effectiveness of Tibetan medical practices. The efficacy of Tibetan remedies for treating arteriosclerosis has already been scientifically proven, and there have been countless confirmations that the hepatitis treaments work. Numerous chronically sick people, given up as lost cases by orthodox medicine, regularly make the pilgrimage to Dharamsala, among them people suffering from cancer, Aids and hepatitis. No one promises that these patients will be cured, but their physical and mental condition, their immune system and quality of life can all be improved. Not least, they find spiritual support in Tibetan medicine, where spiritual exercises are regarded as an important part of healing.

There are about 2,000 Tibetans living in Switzerland, the largest group outside Asia. Here a small business has been producing two well-researched and standardized Tibetan herbal remedies for the past 30 years (*see page 151*), and it may only be a matter of time before the large pharmaceutical companies follow suit.

The huge increase of interest in Tibetan medicine has led to the establishment of associations promoting Tibetan medical practice all over Europe. Their aim is to make this medical system accessible to Europeans, but they have encountered a number of obstacles under European law.

Many Tibetan doctors now travel around Europe, giving lectures and treating hundreds of patients on their way. Acute cases cannot be treated by this means, however, and there tend to be long waiting lists for an appointment. (See page 155 for a list of organizations that may be able to refer you to a Tibetan doctor.)

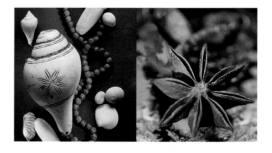

THE ORIGINS OF TIBETAN MEDICINE

A Buddhist art of healing

There is hardly any other widespread system of medicine in which religion plays such an important role as in Tibetan medicine. This deep connection is clear from the fact that Buddhist doctors recite mantras during certain kinds of treatment, and the patient is expected to do likewise.

In former times Mahayana Buddhism, which underpinned the religious rulership of ancient Tibet, was able to spread so successfully in Asia because travelling monk-doctors treated and cured people.

According to the Buddhist view, Tibetan medical knowledge derives from Buddha himself. He propounded medical doctrine in his 'emanation' (his emergence) as Medicine Buddha. The Tibetans revere him as their greatest healer and benefactor, and as 'King of Aquamarine Light', who can overcome all 404 illnesses in a condition of meditative equilibrium. (*See also page 16.*)

The Medicine Buddha and the ideal of compassion

Through the virtue of his compassion, simply by hearing the name of this transcendent, outstanding and perfect comforter and conqueror, whose deeds serve the well-being of all living creatures, we are protected from the agonies of unfortunate life-conditions. I bow down before the Aquamarine Light, the Master of Medicine, the Awakened One, who dissolves the three poisons and the three sufferings.

From the *Root Tantra*

According to Tibetan medicine, the doctor's compassion towards his patient is one of the most important prerequisites for curing illness. In Buddhism the doctor's profession is regarded as noble, since he is obliged to practise the ideal of compassion. The Bodhisattva is viewed as the ideal ethical model for a doctor. This highly evolved being has already attained his goal of enlightenment and could enter Nirvana but chooses through compassion to remain in the world in order to show as many people as possible the path that leads away from suffering.

Before Buddhism

Before Buddhism came to Tibet, a shamanistic medicine and religion called Bon held sway in the snowy Himalayas. Bon was the original religion of the people. It had magical aspects and involved superstition and the summoning of spirits. Vestiges of Bon still remain to this day. In remote mountain regions, in Ladakh for example, the healing traditions of Bon shamans live on. Almost all of these medicine men and women subscribe to the beliefs of Buddhism, and do not find any contradiction between the teachings of Buddha and their magical practice of healing.

According to many texts, the history of Tibetan Buddhism and medicine begins with King Songsten Gampo (AD 620–49), the founder of Greater Tibet. As destiny would have it, this king married two Buddhist princesses – Bhrikuti from Nepal and Weng Cheng from China. They brought the first Buddha statues to these snow-clad mountains, and had temples built in Lhasa. Eventually they converted their husband to their religion, and from then on Buddhism was practised at court.

The new faith met with resistance among the common people. To make this relatively elite doctrine of Buddhism comprehensible, early Buddhists integrated the concepts of Bon with tenets of their own faith. From the very beginning, therefore, Tibetan Buddhism included practices such as exorcism, ritual healings and possessions.

The first medical texts

Under the rule of King Songsten Gampo many texts from Indian literature were translated into Tibetan. There was a lively cultural exchange between India and Tibet and the Chinese princess Weng Cheng is said to have brought a medical text from her homeland that was translated into Tibetan. Songsten Gampo gathered many scholars from India, China and Persia at his court, including doctors, but the king's most outstanding achievement was to develop the Tibetan script. Since this time Tibet's history has been recorded.

In the 8th century King Tisong Detsen (742–98) succeeded in creating a broader base for Buddhism by raising it to the status of national religion in Greater Tibet. It is also thanks to this king that Indian

medical texts were translated into Tibetan for the first time, and these are said to have contributed to the development of Tibetan medicine.

The texts which King Tisong Detsen had collected were very extensive but they were also confusing and sometimes contradictory. His physician, the learned Yuthog Yonten Gonpo the Elder, took it upon himself to make sense of them. Born in 786, Yuthog lived to the age of 125, and is still known as one of Tibet's most famous doctors. Many regarded him as the incarnation of the Medicine Buddha.

Yuthog the Elder journeyed to India three times to learn from doctors there. In order to deepen his understanding of the medical texts, he even arranged a debate between a number of Asian medical experts. Afterwards he interwove the best parts of these texts and created a new whole, which became the original Tibetan doctrine of medicine.

The time was not yet ripe for this knowledge and so the medical texts were concealed so that they might be rediscovered later by the people who were destined to disseminate them. That is why they lay hidden in the Samye monastery for 300 years. The texts were not found again until the 12th century, when they fell into the hands of Yuthog Gonpo the Younger (1126–1212). Like his namesake,

A flower-adorned image of the Buddha stands by the path to the Dharamsala Medical and Astrological Institute. On the right are examples of typical mantra-inscribed stones.

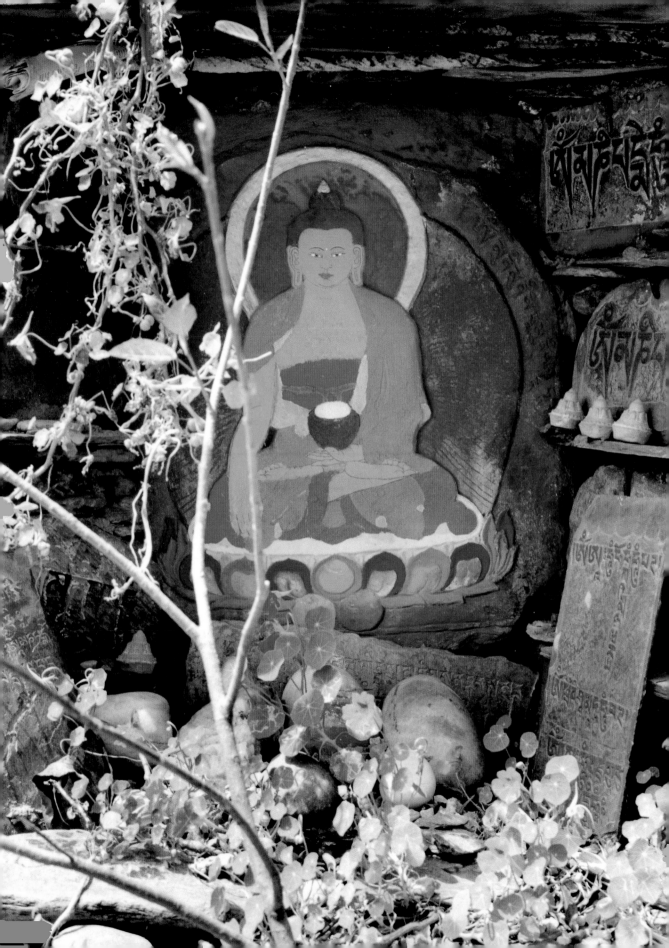

this Yuthog was not only regarded as a great scholar but also as a Tantric master. He probably added to the texts from other sources and adapted them to the needs of the time, creating a medical treatise known as the *Four Tantras*, which even modern researchers have come to describe as a 'magnificent, highly complex work by a Tibetan author of high creative intelligence'.

The Four Tantras

The *Four Tantras* are also known under their Tibetan name of *rGyudbzhi*, which is pronounced (and sometimes written as) 'Gyushi'. It means 'the secret oral tradition of the eight branches of the science of healing'. The *rGyudbzhi* possesses a similar fundamental character to the *Huangdi Neijing* of Chinese medicine, or the *Samhitas* of Ayurvedic medicine. To this day, it is the central work upon which Tibetan medicine is based.

In the *rGyudbzhi*, the Ayurvedic teaching of the threefold nature of bodily energies (the doctrine of the three 'body fluids') is combined with Chinese astrology and teachings about the pulse. The treatise is composed of four separate works, each one of which examines medical knowledge from a different perspective.

The 5th Dalai Lama

Lobsang Gyatso (1617-82), 5th Dalai Lama, is regarded as one of the greatest promoters of Tibetan medicine. During his rule, Tibetan medical practice and culture reached a high point. Under the aegis of the Yellow Church, to which he belonged, the 'Great 5th' re-established Buddhism as the national religion and ordered that Tibet should once more become centrally ruled, which it had not been for a long time.

This Dalai Lama was particularly interested in the *Four Tantras*. He commissioned a new block-printed edition of the texts, and promoted the manufacture of the 'jewel' or 'precious' pills described in them.

He was keen to clarify the still-disputed origin of the *Four Tantras*. He used his authority to support the view that the Buddha Shakyamuni had proclaimed this medicine in India towards the end of his life, by taking the form of the 'Master of Remedies'. Many fundamentalist Buddhist doctors and scholars adhered to this belief right up to the 21st century. The work itself states that it is a translation from Sanskrit of the teachings of the 'Master of Remedies Buddha'.

This Buddha bears the name Bhaishaiyaguru (the radiant king) because healing rays emanate from him. He is almost always portrayed in a blue-green aquamarine colour and is also known as Vaidurya – King of Aquamarine Light. Over the centuries, seven further Buddhas joined the Medicine Buddha. Their common distinguishing feature is that they carry a branch or fruit of the myrobalan tree in their right hand.

A Tibetan medical text from the Four Tantras. *The valuable pages are copied for everyday use.*

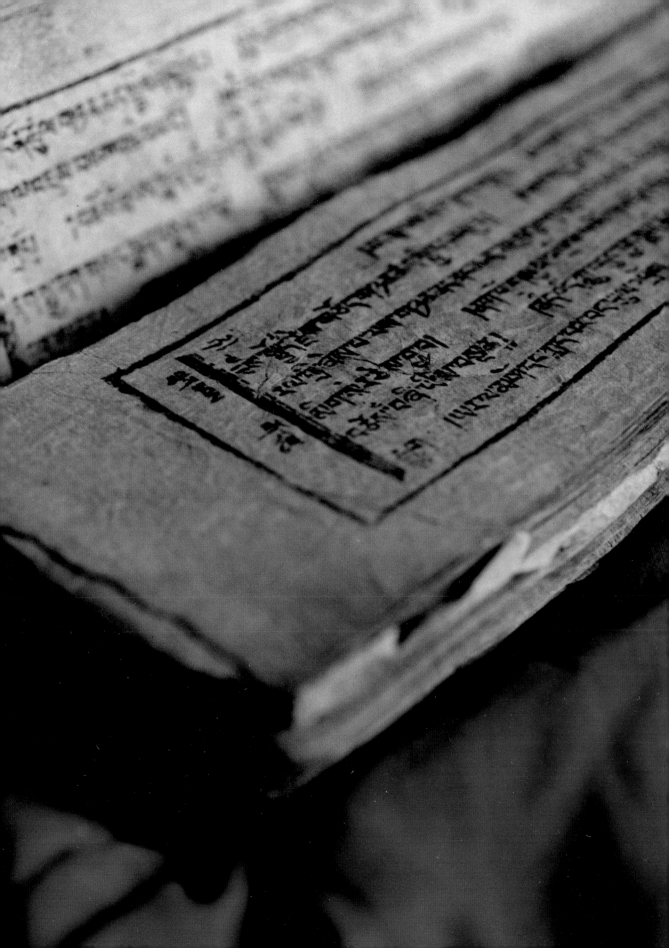

The 5th Dalai Lama appointed his spiritual son Sangye Gyamtso (1653–1705) as his regent, to assume rule until the next Dalai Lama took office. This extremely learned man continued the work of his master in an ambitious and perfectionist manner. His efforts culminated in a new version of the *Four Tantras*. He also added to it his famous commentary, known as the *Blue Beryl*, making it more comprehensible to posterity. This new edition and its commentary have been the foundation of Tibetan medicine ever since. Medical students still spend most of the first four years of their study learning the *Four Tantras* by heart.

The content of the Four Tantras

The first tantra is the *Root Tantra*. It presents teachings about illness and relates all the elements of these teachings to one another in logical sequence. The commentary that accompanies this is illustrated in the second medical scroll picture (*see page 23*), depicting a tree with two trunks. One symbolizes the branches of human physiology, the other the categories of illness. The *Root Tantra* also describes the causes of illness and methods of diagnosis and treatment.

The second tantra is the *Tantra of Enlightenment*. This contains teachings about the body, diagnosis, treatment and medical ethics. There are descriptions of conception and pregnancy, the development of the foetus, of anatomy, physiology, a further classification of illnesses, several chapters on nutrition, the absorption of food, and medicines.

In the third tantra, the *Tantra of Oral Tradition*, also called the *Tantra of Instructions*, all illnesses and their treatments are listed individually, highlighting diagnosis, symptoms and treatment instructions. Sixteen chapters of this longest volume of the four are devoted to the different kinds of fever, while 19 others deal with a variety of illness – from hoarseness to gout, rheumatism and Parkinson's disease. Further chapters are devoted to specialist fields such as gynaecology and paediatrics, while still others deal with poisoning, wounds or fertility treatment. This *Tantra of Oral Tradition* has not yet been translated.

The fourth tantra, also called the concluding tantra or *Latter Tantra*, contains methods of diagnosis, preparation of medicines, methods of treatment and above all secret remedy preparations. This tantra has not yet been translated either.

The 79 Tibetan medicine pictures

Anyone who becomes familiar with Tibetan medicine will discover the intricate and delicate medicine *thangkas*, which are medical scroll pictures on canvas. These master works were commissioned by the regent Sangye Gyamtso to make the *Blue Beryl* as accessible as possible. The 79 *thangkas* present the whole of Tibetan medical teaching in pictorial form and the series is among the greatest achievements of medical iconography. All the images are composed of hundreds of separate vignettes, each of which has a precise textual caption. Each of the 79 *thangkas* is numbered and has its own place in the overall sequence. The series is introduced by a scene showing the Medicine Buddha proclaiming the doctrine of medicine (*see page 57*).

These medicine *thangkas* relate to the various fields of Tibetan medicine – from embryology, anatomy, physiology, methods of diagnosis, materia medica, nutrition and composition of remedies through to all the different forms of treatment.

The Chagpori medical school

Sangye Gyamtso performed another great service when he founded the Chagpori medical school in Lhasa in 1696, in accordance with the wishes of the 5th Dalai Lama who had died ten years previously. The idea was to clarify medical theory and practice in a code of practice. Chagpori was the first national Tibetan medical centre, built in Lhasa on the so-called 'iron hill' close to the Potala palace, the Dalai Lama's winter residence. This centre served as a model for other medical schools founded during the 18th century – in East Tibet, Beijing, Mongolia and Buryat (southern Siberia).

Most of the personal physicians of subsequent Dalai Lamas were trained in Chagpori. Even in the 20th century many of the monk doctors teaching there, and most of the 70 pupils, were monks from the Gelugpa monasteries, known as the 'Yellow Caps'.

Although the Yellow Church was the main proponent of Tibetan medicine, a lay tradition formed alongside this. Teaching Tibetan medicine was no longer a preserve of Buddhist monasteries, and more and more 'worldly' doctors started practising too. They handed down their knowledge within their families from generation to generation, a tradition that is sustained to this day.

The Tibetan Medical and Astrological Institute

Tibetan medicine's systematic adoption by lay doctors began at the time of the 13th Dalai Lama, Tubten Gyatso (1876–1933). In order to provide new impetus for the teaching centre in Chagpori, he founded the Tibetan Medical and Astrological Institute in the centre of Lhasa in 1916, and appointed his personal physician Khyenrab Norbu (1883–1962) to be in charge of it. The Tibetan Medical and Astrological Institute remained the government's medical institute and hospital up to the time of the Chinese invasion. Only half of all medical students came from the monasteries, while the other half were lay students from different regions of Tibet. The institute had the capacity to train up to a hundred students in medicine, astrology and Buddhist teaching at any one time.

The Tibetan Medical and Astrological Institute was destroyed during the Cultural Revolution and not rebuilt until the 1970s. There is more information about this institute on page 132.

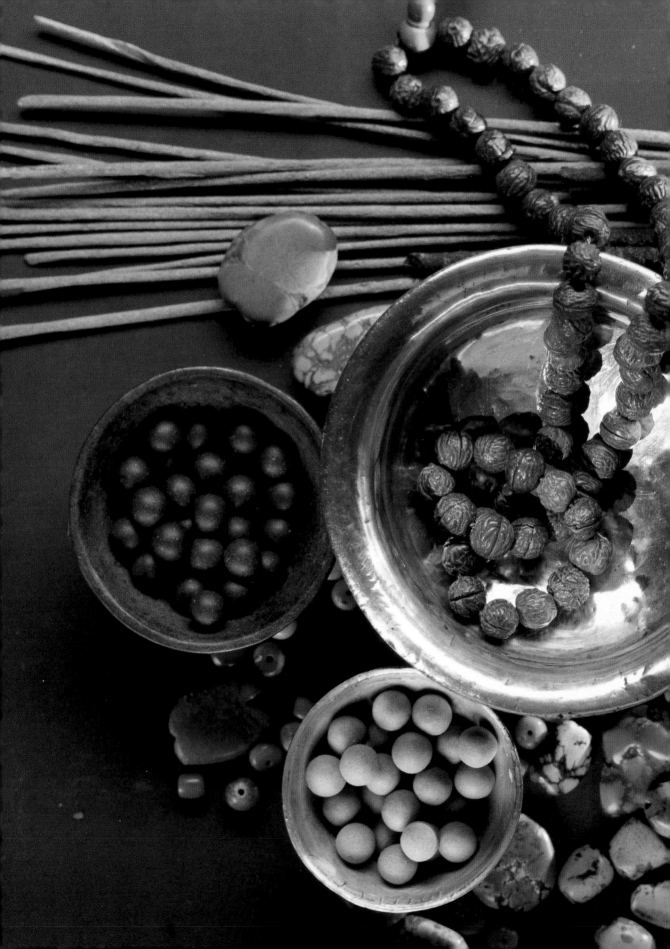

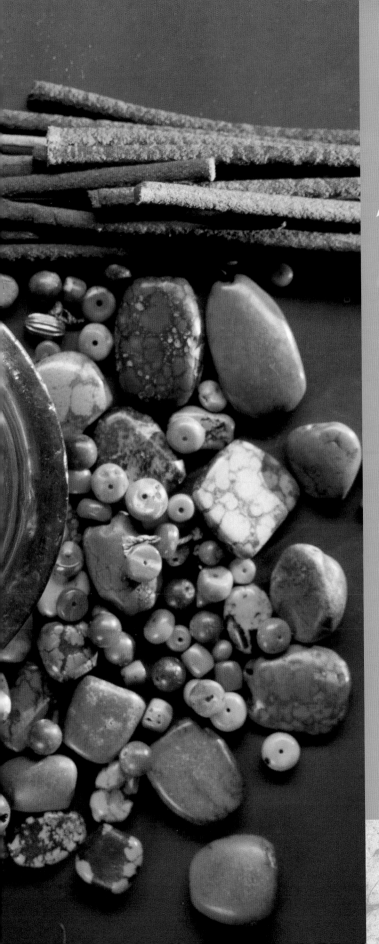

Principles
of
Tibetan
Medicine

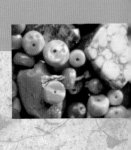

Chapter 2

THE TEACHING OF THE THREE ENERGIES

Like Ayurvedic medicine, Tibetan medicine is based on the teaching of the three body 'juices' or 'fluids'. Wind, bile and phlegm, as they are called in English, are, ideally, in balance and harmony with one another. Lack of balance between them leads to disorders that can result in illness. In contrast to the Greek doctrine of the three humours, the 'fluids' (*nyespa*) of Tibetan medicine are not merely specific bodily substances. It would be wrong to conceive of 'wind' simply as breath or moving air, of 'bile' as the secretion of the gall bladder, and of 'phlegm' as bronchial mucus. Wind, bile and phlegm are symbolic principles which not only relate to the body but also have more rarefied psychological, even spiritual dimensions. To avoid confusion we will use the original Tibetan terms: *rlung* (wind), *mkhrispa* (bile) and *badkan* (phlegm), and refer to them as bodily energies or principles rather than fluids.

The three energies		
English	**Tibetan**	**phonetic**
Wind	*rlung*	loong
Bile	*mkhrispa*	tripa
Phlegm	*badkan*	baekaen

Meaning of the three principles

At a physical level, the three principles refer to bodily energies.

• *rlung* represents the element of movement within the body;
• *mkhrispa* represents the different kinds of warmth in the body;
• *badkan* represents everything of a fluid nature in the body.
These three principles are fundamental ones which apply to all living organisms, including plants and all kinds of animals with which human beings live in harmony.

The three energies also represent physiological principles and are related to the five Tibetan elements of wind, fire, earth, water, space (ether), as well as to the two properties of hot and cold.

Rlung is a dynamic principle belonging to the element of wind, and the central directing principle of our consciousness. *Rlung* is also referred to simply as the life principle, which can intensify the other 'fluids' in both a positive and a negative sense. The *rlung* energy is most active where the nervous system interacts with the hormonal and immune systems and the psyche. This means that all psychosomatic processes in the body are directed by the *rlung* principle. *Rlung* is fundamentally neither hot nor cold, but neutral.

Mkhrispa, in contrast, is related to the element of fire and to the energetic life

Opposite – the Medicine Tree, the 'root of physiology and pathology', depicted on the medicine thangka *number 2, symbolizes the many specific details of health, diagnosis and illness. The lower branch of the left-hand trunk shows the three bodily energies in their healthy state.* Rlung *is depicted as blue,* mkhrispa *yellow, and* badkan *white.*

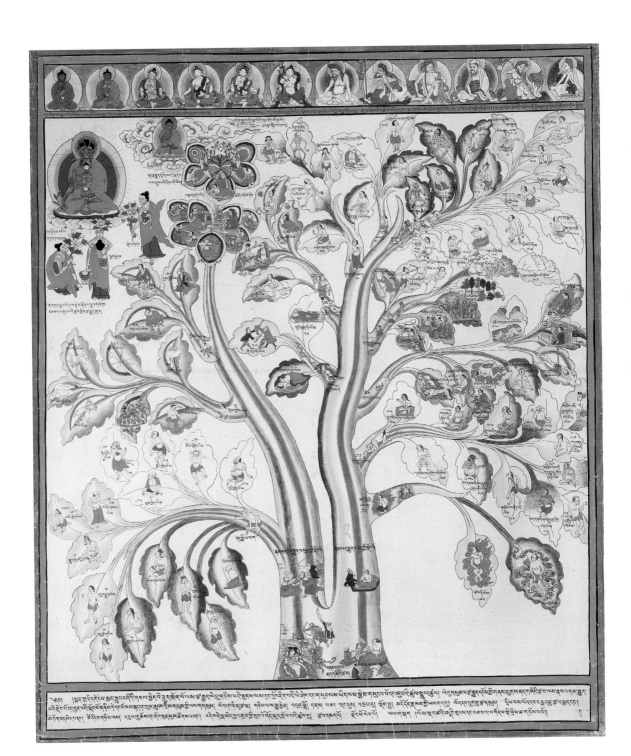

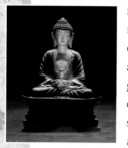

force. This principle is responsible for all processes of dissolution and combustion, so at the purely physical level it governs metabolic and digestive processes. The spiritual qualities ruled by *mkhrispa* include courage, persistence and intelligence; and it possesses the property of warmth or heat.

Badkan combines the two elements of water and earth, and represents the regulation of bodily fluids. All fluid and material aspects of the body, such as lymph or mucus membranes, are influenced by the *badkan* principle. It is related to coldness.

Rlung
the energy of movement

In a healthy person, *rlung* can be found in the lower body. Its task is to coordinate all physical and spiritual activities, as well as the conscious and unconscious, with the help of the nervous system. *Rlung* is also responsible for feelings and the condition of the soul. Breathing, physical strength and sensory perceptions are dependent on *rlung*, as is the pulse and the peristaltic motions of the intestine.

By means of these important functions *rlung* holds the other two energies in balance. The *rlung* energy animates us and directs all biological and soul–mind processes. It is the most important and extensive of the three energies, which is why a *rlung* disorder impairs the body most severely.

Mkhrispa
the fire of life

In a healthy person, *mkhrispa* is found in the body's middle area, and symbolizes all forms of fire – including every process that requires heat to function, such as digestion, assimilation of nutrients and metabolism. *Mkhrispa* is responsible for maintaining body temperature, as well as for the breakdown of substances by combustion. Just as 'inner fire' makes us lively, mentally alert and spirited, it can also provoke rage and over-excitement. In the emotional–psychological area, *mkhrispa* represents action, will, persistence, courage and spiritual clarity. The fire of *mkhrispa* has both destructive and uplifting, life-enhancing qualities, and it is connected with our sense of well-being.

Badkan
the fluid element

Badkan resides in the upper body and symbolizes the fluid element in the human being, as well as stability and weight. Water, *badkan's* main component, controls fluid in our organs and tissue elasticity. The smooth action of our joints depends on this energy. At a spiritual and mental level, *badkan* stands for good memory and ability to concentrate. It is also responsible for deep sleep and strong powers of recuperation. Everything connected with weight and carrying or sustaining is controlled by this principle; and when everything is in order *badkan* creates physical and mental peace.

When one of these energies predominates

The three bodily energies pulsate rhythmically, so their inter-relationship is subject to continual transformations in the healthy body. At certain times of day or at certain seasons, but also at certain times of life, one of the energies will predominate. Sometimes a particular energy 'surges' up from its localized seat in the body, thus creating an imbalance.

TEACHINGS ABOUT ILLNESS

In the *Four Tantras* about 84,000 disorders are referred to, which can cause 404 illnesses. Of these, 101 illnesses are karmically determined and, if untreated, will be fatal. A further 101 illnesses derive from lifestyle and can be healed with the right medicines. Another 101 illnesses are caused by spirits, and these include many nervous diseases. The last 101 illnesses are of a superficial kind, and can be healed by the correct attitude and behaviour.

How the three energies become imbalanced

According to Tibetan medicine, a disorder occurs when the three bodily energies become imbalanced. One or more energies are impaired in their functions at their seat in the body. A good Tibetan doctor can ascertain this 'functional disturbance' simply by taking the patient's pulse. It is essential to get rid of the cause of the disorder, because otherwise the surging energy 'boils over' and spreads to other areas of the body where it does not belong, and the symptoms of disease develop. An overpowering *rlung* energy usually manifests as a 'cold' illness, too much *mkhrispa* engenders 'heat' illnesses, and excessive *badkan* energy leads to 'cold' illnesses.

The classification into cold and hot illnesses

The classification of illnesses and their remedies according to heat and cold is one of Tibetan medicine's most fundamental principles, upon which all other inter-relationships depend. Like the three energies, illnesses have hot and cold characteristics: *mkhrispa* is hot like the sun, as are its corresponding disorders; *rlung* and *badkan* are by nature cold, and related to the moon, so the disorders and illnesses connected with these principles tend to be cold. Yet while *badkan* is clearly cold, the *rlung* principle is harder to grasp, for it can also be categorized as neutral. Since *rlung* is involved in all dynamic processes (of both health and illness), it can intensify both *mkhrispa* and *badkan* disorders. At the onset of every illness, it is the *rlung* principle that alters the level of a bodily energy – in other words the *rlung* principle is always involved in a loss of balance between the three energies.

Whether an illness is hot or cold in nature indicates the therapy that is needed.

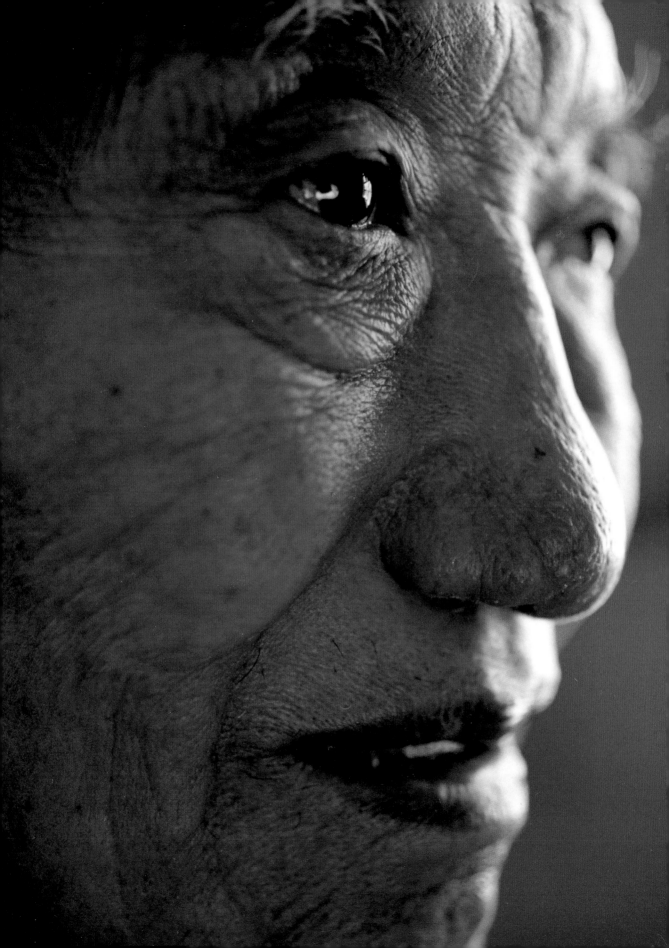

Cold illnesses require hot remedies and treatments, while hot illnesses need cold remedies and treatments.

Simple and combined illnesses

As well as hot and cold illnesses, Tibetan medicine also distinguishes between simple and combined illnesses. In simple illnesses, only one of the three energies is out of balance, while combined illnesses involve a disturbance of two or all three energies. But in treating disease the practitioner should never merely reduce or strengthen the disturbed bodily energies, for this would lead to an imbalance of the other energies and a new, secondary illness would result. In the case of combined illnesses, which are often caused by wrong treatment, the remedy must be a balanced one, possessing both hot and cool active forces. To achieve this, additional balancing substances are always used to complement the medicine and diet prescribed by the doctor.

The seat of illnesses

In Tibetan teachings illnesses have a particular seat in the body and specific symptoms.

Badkan illnesses are situated in the brain and the body's upper region. They relate to the digestive tract, flesh, fat, bone

Monk doctor Tenzin Choedrak, the Dalai Lama's personal physician.

marrow, sperm/egg, faeces, urine, nose, tongue, lungs, spleen, stomach, kidneys and bladder. Characteristic of these illnesses is a continuous sense of feeling cold, weak and lacking in energy. People with *badkan* disorders are constantly tired and weary, and need to sleep a good deal. They often feel unwell after eating. Another typical symptom is water retention in the eyelids, and swollen ankles and wrists. Many patients have congested bronchial tubes or chronically blocked sinuses, and have a tendency to bronchial asthma or chronic coughing. People with *badkan* illnesses often tend to be overweight and mentally sluggish.

Mkhrispa disorders are focused in the centre of the body and in the diaphragm area. They affect blood and sweat, the eyes, liver, gall bladder and the small intestine. Typical *mkhrispa* illnesses are accompanied by fever, and often acute infections or inflammations. Eye infections, boils and other suppurating skin disorders are also typical. Such patients feel 'hot' and are very thirsty, they sweat a lot and their perspiration has a strong odour. Sometimes the eyes have a yellowish tinge.

Rlung disorders are located from the hips downwards. They affect bones, ears, nerve endings, the heart, digestive tract and large intestine. Specific *rlung* complaints include dizziness and tinnitus, tension headaches, poor concentration, tension in the neck, high blood pressure and chronic intestinal disorders such as irritable bowel, bloating, and constipation or diarrhoea. *Rlung* types have a tendency to cold hands and feet, are often tired and at the same time unable to sleep, as well as nervous and talkative. Their mind seems restless, they cannot collect their thoughts and their opinions often 'follow each change of wind'. *Rlung* types worry a lot, often grumble and suffer from general, unspecified anxieties. All in all, *rlung* disorders are often what we in the West term psychosomatic complaints.

The three mind poisons

Tibetan doctors believe that every loss of balance between the three energies is caused by the three spirit poisons. Buddha described these mind poisons as the origin of all suffering. They are ascribed to the energies as follows:
• Greed (desire or attachment) – *rlung*
• Hate (aggression or envy) – *mkhrispa*
• Blindness (ignorance or suppression) – *badkan*

Greed – the illness of desire
Rlung illnesses arise from the energy of greed or craving. In general terms this refers to eternal longings, to craving and desire which continually drive us to want something different or more than we have. But no sooner have we gained what we want than the next wish surfaces. The lust for power and possession is based on an illusion that attaining our heart's desire will make us happy. People believe that possession will help to curb the desire for still more, yet the opposite is the case. The more someone is attached to a craving, for instance, piling possession on possession, the more they become a slave to it.

Hate – the illness of aggression
Mhkrispa illnesses arise from the energy of hatred. Fundamentally this means hatred for all that we cannot have for ourselves. People who cannot satisfy their craving quickly grow aggressive towards those who have more than they do. At such moments they often have feelings of envy, which combine elements of greed and aggression. These gnawing feelings allow them no peace and eat away at the strength of even the strongest characters.

Blindness – the suffering of ignorance
Badkan illnesses arise from blindness or ignorance. However this is not just a question of stupidity, but a refusal to see things as they are. We refuse to accept realities and instead pursue illusions and wishful thinking. To the category of ignorance belongs the illusory idea that man is the focus and centre of the world, for this can lead to selfish and self-seeking behaviour. Thus *badkan* also stands for lethargy and stagnation. The egotist grows rigid with inflexibility if he no longer strives for a living relationship with his surroundings.

Wrong thinking makes you sick
The concept of the three mind poisons demonstrates that a wrong attitude to life – Tibetans call it 'wrong thinking' – should be seen as the cause of every illness. Tibetans regard our basic spiritual outlook on life as the decisive factor for health and illness. For some years now, this ancient Buddhist idea has met with great interest in Western 'mind–body' research. The

modern scientific field of psycho-neuroimmunology – research into the relationship between body and mind – demonstrates ever more clearly that our powers of self-healing are very dependent not only on our attitude to life but also on our ways of thinking.

First remedy: the dharma

The *dharma* is defined as 'the doctrine of universal truth common to all individuals, as proclaimed by the Buddha . . . the moral and religious law that governs individual conduct.' The Buddhist patient will naturally try to overcome his wrong thinking by practising the Buddhist religion. The *dharma* is the first remedy against wrong thinking, which is the first cause of illness.

Further causes of illness are:

- wrong diet
- bad climatic conditions
- bad karma
- unfavourable influence of the stars
- spirits and demons

Illnesses caused by diet

After wrong thinking, wrong diet is the second most important cause of illness, and changing eating habits is the second most important remedy. Only when this proves ineffective will the doctor prescribe a medicine or other therapeutic measure.

According to a Tibetan saying, 'There is no need for medicines if you eat the

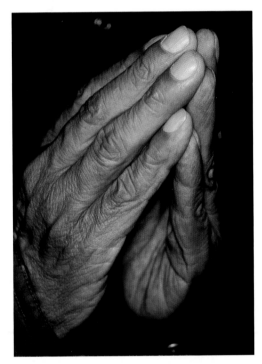

correct diet; but if you do not nourish yourself properly, pills won't make you healthy.'

This is why the Tibetan doctor gives his patient dietary advice at every consultation, quite separately from any other treatment he prescribes. We will examine the importance of medicine and nutrition more closely in Chapter 3.

Illnesses caused by climate

Each constitutional type is suited to particular climatic conditions (*see pages 76-83*) and the elements can be unbalanced by exposure to too much hot or cold weather. They are connected with the seasons, so that some elements become stronger in spring, some in summer, some in autumn and some in winter, and the doctor will have to take this into account.

Illnesses caused by karma

Frequently illnesses occur that seem to have no apparent cause. Tibetan medicine believes that such sufferings arise from the deeds of a former life. It speaks of karmically determined diseases, which include minor ailments as well as cancer, leprosy and epilepsy. If a doctor diagnoses such a complaint, he will 'refer' the patient to a spiritual teacher, a lama. Some illnesses respond very well to religious practices such as rituals or exercises taught by the lama. This therapy is particularly valuable for people who are subject to strong passions such as greed, hatred and blindness. Spiritual instruction may be able to prevent them performing negative deeds, which will become the cause of illness in a future life.

Unfavourable influence of the stars

Even if a doctor can't see a patient face to face, he can understand something about his or her condition after learning their astrological details. Astrology plays a crucial role in the diagnosing and treatment of disease, and also the production of Tibetan medicines (*see page 74*).

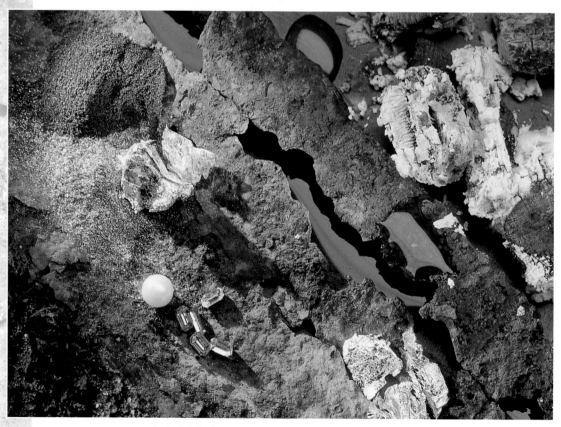

Elements and substances that are used in the manufacture of 'precious pills': earth, water, pearls, diamonds, gold, silver, copper and iron. The metals and precious stones are detoxified in complex alchemical processes.

Illnesses caused by demons

In Tibetan medical teachings, bad spirits are regarded as a disease-inducing factor. Illnesses caused by spirits include severe mental disturbances, as well as gout and tumours. Nagas, or water spirits, the cause of mental 'blindness', supposedly block the 'subtle body energy', by which information is transmitted between physical, mental and emotional planes (*see page 53* for a further explanation of this very important concept). They are also held responsible for swellings and tuberculosis. A lama is called in to treat such illnesses. He will prescribe religious exercises that purify the spirit. The chief aim of these is to develop an altruistic and non-violent attitude, with which the patient can help themselves and the community around them.

THE TIBETAN CLASSIFICATION SYSTEM

The teaching is based on the fact that outer nature and the human organism are both formed of the same basic elements. We take in outer elements through what we eat; and our diet should be so composed that the elements correspond to one another in mutual interrelationship, and that we only ingest what is required by the inner elements of the organism.

Tenzin Choedrak

Tibetan doctors follow a complex yet strictly logical classification system when diagnosing illness and choosing treatments, curative diets and medicinal herbs. Each element has certain characteristics that can be found in bodily energies, nutrition and medicinal plants. Those who know these properties hold the key to therapy.

The following are the most important fundamental aspects of the Tibetan classification system.

The five elements

Of the five elements – earth, water, fire, air and space – only four play a role in the classification of illnesses: air (or wind), fire, water and earth. Since these elements are contained in the three bodily energies, their imbalance also affects the equilibrium of the three 'fluids'. The four elements relate to the following bodily energies and their properties:

Elements	Bodily Energy	Property
Air	*rlung*	neutral (cold)
Fire	*mkhrispa*	hot
Water, earth	*badkan*	cold

The five constituent elements correspond to the following parts of the human body:

Flesh, bones, fat	*earth*
Blood and all bodily fluids	*water*
Body heat	*fire*
Breathing, nervous system	*air*
Cavities in the body	*space*

The eight active forces and the seventeen qualities

Each element also has eight 'active forces' (*nuspa*) and seventeen 'qualities' (*yontan*).
• The eight active forces are: heavy, oily, cool, dull, light, harsh, hot, sharp
• The seventeen qualities are: heavy, stable, dull, dry, fluid, cool, hot, sharp, oily, harsh, light, supple, pale, cold, gentle, smooth, flexible.

The seventeen qualities are attributed to the five elements, as follows:

Earth	Water	Fire	Air	Space
heavy	fluid	light	light	empty, penetrates everything
stable	cool	hot	mobile	
dull	dull	sharp	cold	
oily	gentle	harsh	harsh	
gentle	heavy	oily	dry	
dry	oily	mobile	pale	
smooth	supple	dry		
counteracts				
rlung disorders	*mkhrispa* disorders	*badkan* disorders	*mkhrispa-badkan* disorders	

The six taste spheres

In order to know which elements compose a food or medicinal plant, it is essential to recognize its 'taste sphere' (known in Tibetan as *ro*). There are six tastes: sour, salty, sharp, sweet, bitter and astringent (or 'contracting'). Each of these taste spheres is based on certain elements. What is important in choosing the right medicinal plant are the active forces that arise from the combination of various elements in the plant.

How the eight active forces influence the energies
• Heavy diminishes *rlung* and increases *badkan*
• Oily diminishes *rlung* and increases *mkhrispa* and *badkan*
• Cool diminishes *mkhrispa* and increases *rlung* and *badkan*
• Dull diminishes *mkhrispa* and increases *badkan*
• Light diminishes *badkan* and increases *rlung*
• Harsh diminishes *badkan* and increases *rlung*
• Hot diminishes *badkan* and increases *mkhrispa*
• Sharp diminishes *badkan* and increases *mkhrispa*

The six tastes, five elements and eight active forces break down as follows:
• Sour: hot, oily, heavy, sharp, harsh fire, earth
• Salty: oily, harsh, sharp, hot, heavy water, fire
• Sharp: light, harsh, sharp, hot fire, air
• Sweet: heavy, dull, cool, oily water, earth
• Bitter: cool, dull, harsh, light water, air
• Astringent: cool, dull earth, air.

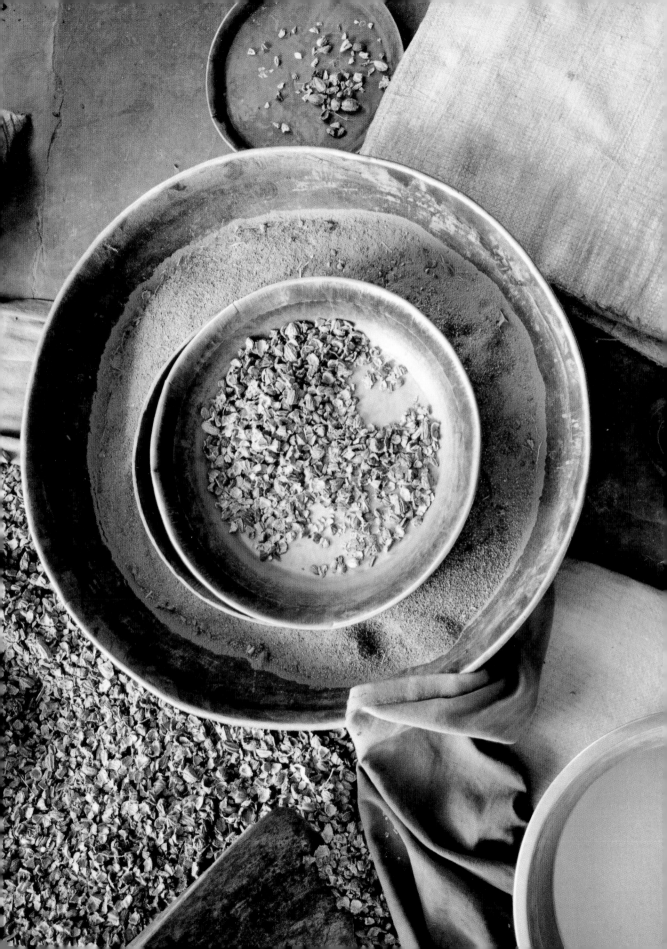

Treatment according to these classifications

Using this schema, a Tibetan doctor can determine the overall effect of a medicinal plant, and administer it in a directed way. As soon as the pulse diagnosis reveals which of the bodily energies are out of balance, the classification system will indicate the elements that are disturbed. For instance, in a *badkan* disorder the elements of water and earth are too pronounced; the taste sphere ascribed to these is sweet, and *badkan* and sweet have the same qualities. A medicinal plant whose taste sphere is sweet would therefore make the illness worse. To cure the disorder, a plant that possesses the opposite active force is required. In this case a plant with the taste sphere of sharp would be right, for it contains the elements opposite to water and earth, those of fire and air.

It takes years of study for Tibetan doctors to grasp the complexity of this classification system. Nevertheless, we can all use it in simplified form to help ourselves choose the right diet. For lay people it is enough to know whether a food or medicinal plant is warming or cooling in its effect, and from this can be deduced its effect on the three bodily energies. Those who know which taste sphere the medicinal plant or food belongs to are able to determine the elements at work in the plant. Therefore it is possible to draw up a dietary programme to balance the individual bodily energies for each person.

METHODS OF DIAGNOSIS

In the *Root Tantra*, the first of the four Tantra volumes, 38 diagnostic procedures for determining an illness are described – yet this is a purely theoretical list. Those who go to a Tibetan doctor nowadays find that three or at most four methods of diagnosis are used: taking the pulse, urine analysis, examination of the tongue and questioning. Sometimes only a single method is enough – the most important one of all, that of pulse diagnosis. The best Tibetan doctors can make a diagnosis by means of the pulse alone.

Pulse diagnosis

Taking the pulse is seen as the mainstay of Tibetan diagnosis, and the doctor will almost invariably turn his attention to this first and foremost. It can seem strange to Westerners that a Tibetan doctor will take their pulse before having a close look at them or asking them any questions. Pulse diagnosis is a highly developed skill, and requires a high degree of sensitivity in the fingertips as well as a great deal of experience and intuition. Some Tibetans claim that Western doctors can never learn the art of pulse-taking in its highest form, because they lack the necessary sensitivity in their fingers. What is certain is that even among Tibetan doctors there are only a few great masters of the skill, for pulse diagnosis is one of the hardest disciplines of Tibetan medicine.

By taking the pulse, a doctor can recognize disorders of very different kinds. He examines the condition of the five vital and six cavity organs, the equilibrium of the three bodily energies and five elements, and the sites of possible disturbances in the upper, middle and lower body. All in all, Tibetan pulse diagnosis is an astonishingly precise procedure, whose results can easily match those of the 'check-up' made by a Western doctor, but without incurring high laboratory and equipment costs because the Tibetan doctor needs only his hands. Many who have experimented by having their pulse taken by several different doctors have been surprised by the uniformity of diagnosis. It is a routine matter to use this method in diagnosing vascular system disorders, such as high blood pressure or diabetes. And most doctors have no difficulty in ascertaining organ weaknesses and the nature of illnesses (for example, *rlung/badkan* disturbances). Even the early stages of cancer can often be diagnosed through the pulse.

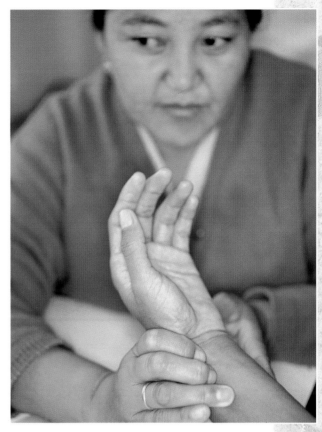

type. There is more information about constitution types and tips for maintaining good health in the next chapter.

Pulse diagnosis and constitution type

Pulse diagnosis is not only used for diagnosing illness. Healthy people can benefit from it, because it helps the doctor to judge precisely which of the seven constitution types they belong to and recommend effective measures they can take to prevent illness. Each constitution type has inherent weaknesses and by adopting certain lifestyle and dietary habits people can ensure that they do not fall prey to the illnesses likely to affect their

What to avoid the day before a pulse diagnosis

There are particular rules the patient must observe the day before a pulse diagnosis. If they do not, the doctor may send them home again because the pulse is 'too agitated' and therefore little can be read from it. These rules are especially important if the doctor does not already know a patient.

On the day before a pulse diagnosis, the patient should avoid all extremes, behave normally and they should not consume strong tea, alcohol or too much yoghurt. They should avoid unusual or extreme exertion, as well as sexual intercourse and sleeping during the day. On the day of the diagnosis, they should not drink any coffee and if possible, they should come well-rested to an early-morning appointment.

If it is impossible for the patient to attend an early-morning appointment, perhaps because they are travelling from far away, then the doctor will urge them to rest a little before the consultation, so that the pulse can calm down.

Each finger senses two organs

The pulse is taken on the radial artery at the wrist. The doctor places his index, middle and ring fingers on the pulse. The index finger presses only on the skin, the middle finger presses through to the muscle, and the ring finger as far as the bone. With a male patient the doctor should take the pulse by placing his own right hand on the man's left wrist; and vice versa with a female patient – at least in theory. In practice the doctor usually takes the pulse of the hand nearest to him. Each of his fingers senses two organs. The doctor 'reads' them with two parts of his fingertips. The upper part of the fingertip senses a vital organ, the lower part senses a cavity or vessel organ (such as intestine or stomach). The doctor is also able to diagnose the condition of upper, middle and lower body.

• The index finger senses lungs and large intestine, heart and small intestine, as well as the upper body and the element of fire.

• The middle finger senses the liver and gall bladder, spleen and stomach, as well as the middle region of the body and the element of earth.

• The ring finger senses left and right kidneys, bladder, testicles or the female reproductive organs, as well as the lower body and the element of water.

Pulse diagnosis for men

	RIGHT WRIST	LEFT WRIST
Upper body	heart, small intestine	lungs, large intestine
Middle body	spleen, stomach	liver, gall bladder
Lower body	right kidney, testicles	left kidney, bladder

Pulse diagnosis for women

	RIGHT WRIST	LEFT WRIST
Upper body	heart, small intestine	lungs, large intestine
Middle body	liver, gall bladder	spleen, stomach
Lower body	right kidney, bladder	left kidney, womb

For female patients, the doctor takes the pulse on the other side from men. The reason is because in Tibetan embryology, the heart forms in a different position depending on whether the child is male or female. When taking a child's pulse, the doctor will feel the veins in the ears instead of the wrist.

Once the doctor has assessed the condition of the organs, he is able to diagnose *rlung*, *mkhrispa* and *badkan* illnesses. Pulses are determined by constitution, and each of them stands for one of the three bodily energies. The constitution pulses have characteristic properties classified as male, female or neutral (though these designations have nothing to do with sexual characteristics). The male pulse is similar to the *rlung* principle, the female to the *mkhrispa* and the neutral to the *badkan* principle. Yeshi Donden, formerly personal physician to the Dalai Lama, who now has his own practice in Dharamsala, ascribes the following properties to the pulses:

– male (*rlung*): full, coarse
– female (*mkhrispa*): fine, quick
– neutral (*badkan*): steady, slow, soft

Yeshi Donden makes the following observations about the quality of the pulse, based on his observations:

• 'A man with a fine, quick pulse will live a long time. A woman with a full, coarse pulse will bear children who have accrued positive karma from former lives.'

• A healthy pulse beats five times for each of the doctor's breaths. If there are more pulse beats, the illness is classified as hot, and with fewer, the illness is cold.

The few true masters of pulse diagnosis are able to sense almost all of the 43 kinds of pulse. They can detect both acute and chronic illnesses and recognize mental problems by this means. It is said that they can even perceive the influence of spirits. Less advanced healers can only use the pulse to detect whether an illness is hot or cold.

Taking the pulse is an extremely precise method of diagnosis, whose efficacy depends very largely on the doctor's skill.

Unless a doctor is extremely experienced, he shouldn't rely solely on a pulse diagnosis. Particularly in the case of serious illnesses, X-rays and ultrasound scans are recommended.

Urine diagnosis

Tibetans always bring a fresh sample of their morning urine to appointments with their doctor. Urine examination is regarded as the second most important diagnostic tool in Tibetan medicine, and it is particularly important if the pulse diagnosis has been inconclusive. Many doctors examine the urine of each new patient on principle, to guide their diagnosis. If the doctor already knows a patient, urine analysis is only used where there is some doubt about the cause of the problem.

In practical terms, a urine diagnosis is a fairly quick procedure. The doctor goes to the toilet bowl or a sink and pours the patient's urine into a small white bowl or a beaker. Then he stirs up the urine to a foam, rather like beating egg-white. A simple stick is used for stirring; Yeshi Donden uses a small bamboo whisk. The type and size of the bubbles that form as froth indicate the patient's condition. The colour, smell, the rising steam and the albumen content (a cloudy substance in the urine) are further diagnostic criteria.

The perfect urine

There is a description of urine analysis in the *Four Tantras*, but Yeshi Donden's comments are more relevant to our own times:

'The urine of a healthy person is by and large the bright, cheerful yellow of "Dri" butter (from a female yak). The smell is similar to the cream that collects on the surface of milk. The steam is neither too strong nor too weak, there is neither much nor little of it, and the time it takes until the urine cools to the point of emitting no steam is neither especially long nor short. The bubbles or froth are not particularly remarkable – neither very large nor very small. The bubbles are neither long nor short, nor very small, but rather an average foam on the surface of the urine.'

The triple urine examination

Ideally patients should provide urine which they have passed between four and five in the morning. They should collect the mid-stream urine, rather than the initial flow. In theory the urine is examined three times: first while it is still warm, then when it is lukewarm, and finally after it has cooled. On the first examination, colour, steam, smell, bubbles and froth are investigated; at the second, the albumen and chylus (a fatty substance that rises to the surface) are examined; finally the duration of colour changes is noted, and other changes recorded.

In urine analysis, there is a great divergence between theory and practice, for the stipulations of the *Four Tantras* cannot usually be fulfilled. Few patients will find a doctor prepared to examine their urine at dawn. That is only likely to be possible in hospital or for high-ranking personalities such as the Dalai Lama, who have their own personal physicians. Most people would find it difficult to deliver their urine before eight in the morning, and normally it will have cooled by the time the patient is seen, for doctors' practices are particularly busy in the morning. The following method of urine testing can be performed by the patient and the results passed on to the doctor:

• Warm urine: note the colour, steam, smell, bubbles and foam
• Lukewarm urine: look for signs of albumen and chylus
• Cold urine: note the length of time colour changes persist.

As with the pulse diagnosis, a patient should observe certain rules the day before a urine analysis: avoid extremes, don't drink strong tea or alcohol, and don't eat too much yoghurt, which would affect the urine colour. He or she should not have sexual intercourse during the night before analysis.

Interpretation of symptoms

The *Root Tantra* describes symptoms in brief:
• *rlung* illnesses: the urine is watery, with large bubbles;
• *mkhrispa* illnesses: the urine is reddish-yellow, unpleasant smelling, and gives off a lot of steam;
• *badkan* illnesses: the urine is whitish, with little smell or steam.

However, this outline only describes straightforward illnesses relating to a single

Medicine thangka number 54 illustrates pulse diagnosis. The upper section shows preparation, the middle shows techniques, and the bottom depicts the time of year, cycle of the moon and other factors.

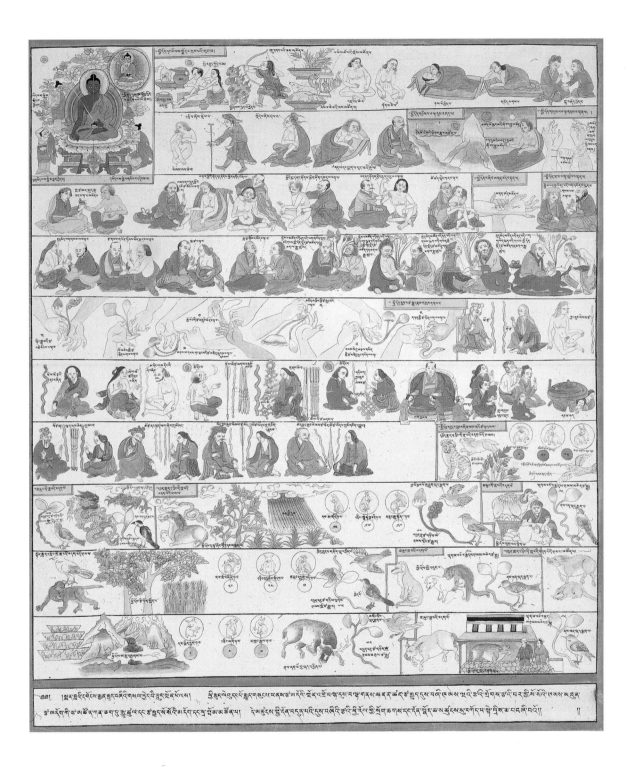

bodily energy. Things become significantly more complex in the case of hot–cold combinations, which show the characteristics of both types of illness – for instance, when the urine has a pale bluish colour, characteristic of a cold illness, and at the same time a thick albumen skin, which is the sign of a hot illness. This would indicate a combined slight cold illness and severe hot illness. In such cases, the patient should definitely consult a doctor.

Tongue diagnosis

Tongue diagnosis is relatively imprecise and is only used to complement other diagnostic methods. Tongue symptoms are described as follows in the *Root Tantra*:
• *rlung* illnesses: red, dry, rough
• *mkhrispa* illnesses: thick, coated in a pale-yellow mucus
• *badkan* illnesses: thick, pale coating, dull, smooth, moist.

Questioning

Before the doctor takes a patient's pulse, he will have formed a general impression of his or her appearance. Western patients will find the Tibetan approach unfamiliar. For example, it is common for the doctor to tell the patient about the complaints he is likely to have, rather than the other way round. Tibetan doctors do not expect the patient to explain why they have come. However, many Tibetan doctors practising in the West have now adopted Western ways and will at least ask the reason for the consultation.

Once the doctor has diagnosed an illness, he will next try to discover its causes. By questioning the patient, he can find out whether the disorder has arisen through direct causes such as wrong diet or behaviour. Such causes result in quite specific complaints, which he will ask about.

Symptoms of direct causes of illness of the *rlung* type are, for instance, shivering or chill, transient, unspecific pains in the hips, thighs and joints, mental instability and hunger pangs.

Mkhrispa illnesses give rise to a bitter taste in the mouth, headaches, pains in the upper body and after digestion.

Badkan illnesses are accompanied by lack of appetite, digestive disorders with vomiting, flatulence, an internal and external sense of coldness, and feeling unwell after eating.

If the patient confirms these symptoms, it is a fairly sure sign of wrong diet or behaviour. The wrong diet in Tibetan medicine means food that does not correspond to your bodily energy type.

Here are a few examples of types of behaviour that give rise to disturbances of the three bodily energies:
• *rlung* illnesses are encouraged by fasting.
BENEFICIAL: relaxing in a warm, shaded and unrestrictive environment; do not stay beside large lakes or at the seaside; do not climb trees.
• *mkhrispa* illnesses are encouraged by sitting in hot sun or in other hot places, and by sudden physical exertion.
BENEFICIAL: staying somewhere cool.

• *badkan* illnesses are encouraged by sitting or sleeping on grass or earth. BENEFICIAL: warm clothing; sitting by a fire or in the sun.

After diagnosis and investigation of the causes, the doctor will choose a method of treatment. In all cases, therapy is complemented by advice on diet and lifestyle. Sometimes this is limited to advising the patient not to bathe in or drink cold water. In other cases, the patient will receive detailed dietary advice and very specific suggestions of ways to change his whole lifestyle, similar to a Western counselling session.

TREATMENT

Treatment that draws on the whole spectrum of Tibetan medicine is a very differentiated and versatile mind–body–spirit therapy. It encompasses all dimensions of existence, and the first and most important remedy of all is to lead a religious life. Beyond that, further therapies relate to nutrition and right conduct, pills and herbal remedies, moxibustion, use of a gold cauterizing rod, cupping, prayers and mantras.

Internal and external therapies

All treatments are divided into three categories:

1 - Internal remedies, which include herbal remedies, laxatives, emetics, inhalations, remedies taken via the nose, and enemas.

2 - External remedies such as massage, mineral baths, incense treatments, bleeding, acupressure, acupuncture, moxibustion with or without golden needles, cupping and cauterizing.

3 - Religious remedies. These include chakra healing, laying-on of hands, meditation, Tibetan curative yoga, bathing exercises, prayers and mantras as well as visualization techniques.

Treatment in everyday practice

As we saw in relation to diagnosis methods, the daily practice of medicine is quite different from the theory. This also applies to treatment. Very busy Tibetan doctors, who may see up to a hundred patients a day, use only a specific, limited spectrum from the treatment options described above. Any further, time-consuming methods, such as massage or baths – if prescribed at all – are delegated to doctors' assistants; and spiritual remedies are the responsibility of lamas.

Basics of Tibetan treatment

In surgeries, therefore, doctors practise the 'basics' of Tibetan medicine. Although these methods are not all-encompassing, they are highly effective. Below are therapies commonly available, listed in order of importance:

• Healing through diet and lifestyle
• Prescribing herb pills and remedies
• Cupping
• Moxibustion with or without golden needles
• Cauterization

Healing through diet and lifestyle

The doctor will initially try to balance out disharmonies between *rlung*, *mkhrispa* and *badkan* by prescribing specific diets, nutrition guidelines and forms of conduct. Only when this fails will he prescribe additional medicines. Tenzin Choedrak, currently one of the Dalai Lama's three personal physicians, says: 'Good nutrition and a good way of life will, according to Tibetan medicine, ensure that circumstances are not created that allow the causes of illness to arise. That is why Tibetan medicine is a gentle, preventive medicine. Balance in diet leads to a balance of the bodily energies.'

Treatment with herbal remedies

A very large proportion of the two hundred or so medicines used by Tibetan doctors are composed of plants and herbs. Only about 20 remedies contain ingredients of animal origin; and in exceptional cases there are 10 minerals that can be added. The famous 'jewel' or 'precious' pills contain pulverized precious and semi-precious stones.

Tibetan herbal remedies also include both expelling remedies – such as laxatives, emetics and enemas (though these are little used nowadays) – and incense treatments (*see page 100*).

When Westerners think of Tibetan medicine, they probably think of herb pills first and foremost. These are classic compounds that can combine up to a hundred different substances.

Manufacturing the pills

Producing herb pills is a great art. After the plants have been collected, they are carefully cleaned and dried, and then cut into pieces with a knife. This preparation often takes several days. The next step is to weigh and mix the substances, and then grind them. Grinding occurs in very different ways according to available technology. In Ladakh, for instance, doctors don't have much equipment, and so they grind the herbs with a stone and sieve the powder through a cloth. Water is carefully added to this herb-flour to produce a porridge-like consistency, which is formed first into sausages and then into balls with the aid of a machine rather like a mincer. To make the balls equally round they are placed in large, shallow bowls that are moved by hand in a rhythmic, circular motion.

In the Tibetan Medical and Astrological Institute in Dharamsala, they use modern machines. The herb mixture is first coarsely and then finely ground, and turned into a powder in mixing drums. The 'pill-turning' also takes place in these drums.

Sometimes – for instance when butter pills are made – the herb ingredients are cooked for days to form a porridge, in

Precious pills are individually wrapped in tissue paper and sealed.

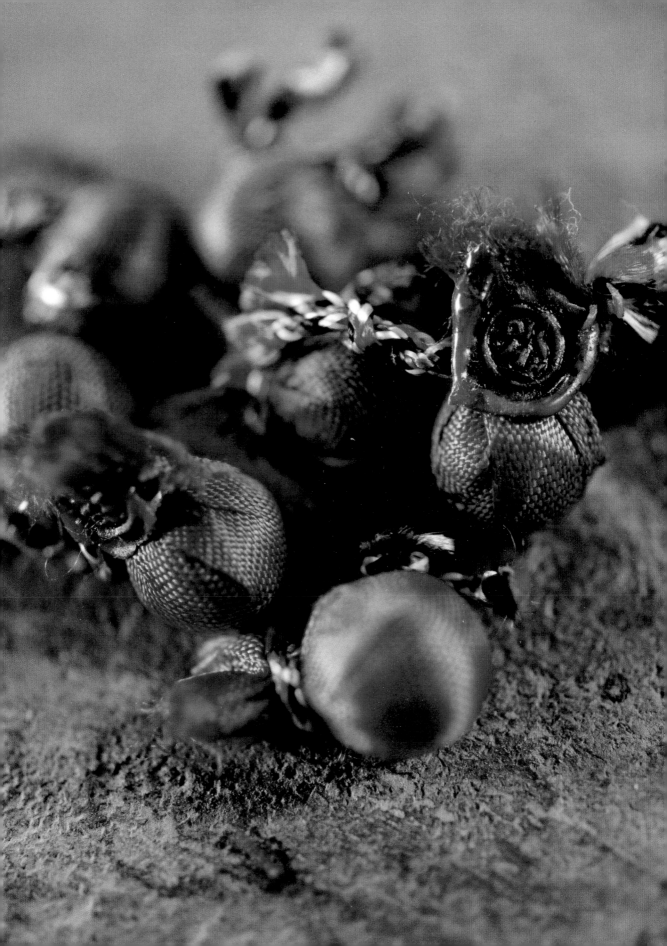

order to potentize the active constituents. Roughly 100kg of medicinal herbs can be reduced to 10kg of active constituent during this process. The mixture is heated and filtered until it can be formed into pills.

Many doctors activate their herbal remedies using the meditative power of mantras. During the gathering of the herbs and before and after manufacture, doctors meditate and visualize themselves and also the pill as a particular deity.

The uses of herb pills

Tibetan pills are prescribed to remedy countless physical complaints. Just to mention a few, they are used in the treatment of stomach and intestinal tract infections, high blood pressure, asthma, thromboses, cataracts, breast and intestinal cancers, and even for dissolving gall and kidney stones. The pills also help alleviate the physical symptoms of psychosomatic *rlung* disorders. Some herb pill treatments take years to work, while others immediately improve the patient's sense of well-being. Pills are usually prescribed for four weeks at a time, after which the patient is invited to return to ascertain if the therapy has been effective.

Magical jewel pills

Jewel pills are of a very special nature. In English they are also known as 'precious pills', because they contain gold, silver and precious stones. Their magical fame is partly due to the costly, extremely complex

and difficult process of manufacture, which is linked to specific alchemical and astrological conditions. For instance, these pills are never allowed to see the light of day. They must be made in the dark, by candlelight, and ingested under the same conditions. Precious pills are individually stored in tissue paper and – those that come from the Tibetan Medical and Astrological Institute, at least – sealed with a monogram seal. In comparison to other herb pills, precious pills are expensive, costing the equivalent of about £3 sterling each.

Many sick people put their last hope in these pills when Western medicine can't help them. Large numbers of people suffering from Aids and cancer come to Dharamsala from all over the world to consult doctors there, and to be treated with precious pills. These medicines are also used prophylactically, to maintain health, for they help sustain the equilibrium of the elements. In some acute cases they have been known to have very rapid effects.

The *Kalachakra Tantra*, proclaimed by the Shakyamuni Buddha, author of the *Four Tantras*, predicts the terrible chemical and radiation pollution of our times. Precious pills are very important in the treatment of illnesses that arise as a result. Following the nuclear disaster at Chernobyl, Tenzin Choedrak travelled to see the people who had fallen ill there and offered his help. As he reports, the symptoms of radiation sickness were low blood pressure, fever, swollen glands, itchy eyes, pains in the bones and a burning feeling all over the body. He prescribed precious pills to ease the victims' suffering, primarily 'Rinchen Mang-sByor' and 'Rinchen grang-byor' (*see page 47*) combined with other medicines. Some patients were able to leave hospital after taking these Tibetan medicines. A scientific explanation of their effect might be that they bind radioactive heavy metals with bodily salts, which are then excreted.

Despite shortages of resources and finances, Tenzin Choedrak has made it possible to manufacture eight different kinds of precious pills at the Tibetan Medical and Astrological Institute in Dharamsala. This great master of medicine succeeded in setting up the highly complex mineral and metal detoxification process there, in exile (*see also pages 138-42*). The procedure draws partly on the secret teachings of the *Kalachakra Tantra*, which is only passed on by word of mouth.

Pill-taking rituals

Strict rules must be observed when taking the pills if they are to be fully effective. From the day before taking a pill to a week afterwards, patients must not consume alcohol, meat, fish, eggs, raw fruits, raw vegetables, garlic, anything fried, sharp or sour; they mustn't exert themselves, have sex, cold baths or – something Tibetan medicine generally regards as harmful – sleep during the day.

On the evening before the pill is taken, it is crushed within its wrapping, the powder is poured into a porcelain cup and hot water is added. The cup is then covered with a cloth and left to stand overnight. The patient should not get cold overnight, but should be warmly wrapped in blankets. The best time for taking the pill is five in the morning. Powder and water are stirred clockwise with the ring finger. If necessary, a little hot water can be added to the mixture so that it is not too cold. After taking the mixture the patient should drink a glass of warm, boiled water and lie relaxing and sweating in bed for an hour. Buddhists recite the following mantra as they do so: *tadyatha aum bhaishiya bhaishya maha bhaishya raja samud gate svaha*.

The eight precious pills

The Tibetan Medical and Astrological Institute in Dharamsala issues information leaflets about the precious pills, which list their ingredients and the illnesses for which they are prescribed. The following information comes from these leaflets. The names of the pills, taken from Tibetan script, can be found in the Tibetan Medical and Astrological Institute museum.

Rinchen Ichags-ril Chen-mo
The Great Precious Iron Pill

The great precious iron pill contains 40 ingredients, including iron filings, three myrobalans without seeds, Kashmir saffron, musk, hardened elephant bile, purified magnetic ironstone and naturally occurring mineral asphaltum.

It is prescribed for all eye complaints such as conjunctivitis, cataracts,

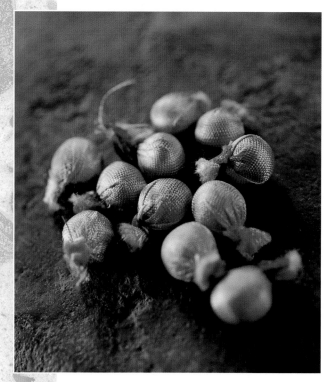

Rinchen Gyu-rNying-25
The Great Precious Old Turquoise 25

This consists of 25 ingredients including old turquoise, coral and pearls that have been detoxified. It also contains purified iron filings, alsphatum, *Crocus sativus L.*, musk, three myrobalans without seeds, two types of sandalwood, *Eugenia caryophyllata (thumb)*, *Saxicus pasumensis marg.* and *Adhatoda vasica.*

The turquoise pill is cold by nature. It is suitable for all liver disorders, relieves a sense of pressure in the upper body, eases neck stiffness, headache, nose-bleeds, bloodshot eyes, pains in the armpits and loss of appetite from an upset stomach. It heals a liver damaged by alcohol abuse or food poisoning.

Rinchen btso-bKru Dha-shel Chen-mo
The Great Precious Purified Moon Crystal

This pill is derived from a 15th-century recipe and combines 50 different ingredients, including gold, silver, copper, brass, lead and bronze, which are detoxified before being processed with the vegetable ingredients. At least two people are needed to manage the detoxification procedure: solutions are added to the metals and then they are boiled, sieved and distilled. The gold alone has to distil for 54 hours.

The plant constituents are: *Gynachum forresti, Sauurea lappa Clarke, Commiphora molmol Engl., Strychnos nux-vomica L., Myristica fragrans Houtt.*, and *Eugenia caryophyllata (thumb).*

The Moon Crystal pill is an antidote to toxic conditions. It purifies the blood and

over-sensitivity to light, bloodshot eyes, softening of the optic nerve, irritation from foreign bodies in the eye, swollen eyelids caused by wind, swellings and pustules of the eye, eye irritations caused by a disorder of the tear ducts, inflammation of the tear ducts, weeping and over-dry eyes, uncontrollable blinking, and generally for maintaining the health of all blood vessels. This pill is also used for eye disorders caused by food poisoning, illnesses caused by blood impurities in the liver, and for patients who are coughing up blood because of stomach ulcers.

In addition to the Medicine Buddha's mantra (*see page 51*), the mantra 'Om Mani Padme Hum' should be recited several times before taking the pill.

regenerates blood circulation, heals stomach ulcers and liver disease, eases pains caused by sudden change of diet or climate. It is good for treating hair loss, intermittent fever and post-viral conditions. It fights infections and cures illnesses caused by excessive eating or alcohol abuse. It is a good tonic for dark-skinned, thin people with a weak constitution. It clears the senses and restores memory. It helps pleurisy, coughing up bloody sputum and mucus discharge. In healthy people, this pill lengthens life expectancy and has a rejuvenating effect.

Ringchen Mang-sByor Chen-mo
The Great Multi Compound Precious Pill

This pill contains around 50 ingredients, including gold, silver and iron, as well as detoxified precious stones like coral and turquoise. Vegetable constituents include: *Saussurea lappa Clarke, Strychnos nux-vomica L., Eugenia caryophyllata (thumb), Areca catechu L.* and nutmeg.

Rinchen Mang-sByor Chen-mo calms all 404 illnesses. It is particularly suitable for complaints where there is any disturbance of the blood, *rlung, mkhrispa* or *badkan* energies. It heals old wounds and throat swellings, is used specifically against food poisoning, insect and animal bites, as well as in illnesses caused by poisonous plants or chemical pollution. It helps against chronic and recurring or intermittent illnesses, various kinds of fever and cases of intestinal and mouth bleeding resulting from severe illnesses. This pill also extends life expectancy for those in good health, as well as protecting people from evil.

Rinchen grang-byor Riln-Nag Chen-mo
The Great Cold Compound Precious Black Pill

This pill is produced in the Tibetan Medical and Astrological Institute following directions in the *Kalachakra Tantra* and using a recipe that comes directly from the 13th century.

In the *Four Tantras* it was prophesied that the people of our century would suffer 18 new kinds of illness, caused by impurities in our food and environment. This precious pill is especially intended for modern times. It contains more than 100 ingredients, including gold, silver, copper and iron, as well as the precious stones sapphire, emerald, turquoise, ruby and diamond, all in detoxified form. In addition it contains a large number of herbs, including *Crocus sativus L.*, silicious bamboo concretion, *Myristica fragrans Houtt., Phytolacca esculenta Van Houtte, Seneciodianthus Franch., Delphinium brunonianum Royle, Oxytropis sp.* and *Berberis aristata D.C.*

This pill is effective against infectious fevers and colic. It stops greying hair and wrinkles and strengthens the bones, combats arthritis and stomach ulcers, ensures physical well-being and clarity of sense impressions. It is helpful in all types of food poisoning, chemical and metal poisoning, and chronic illnesses caused by environmental pollution. This is one of the pills Tenzin Choedrak prescribed for the victims of radiation sickness after the accident in Chernobyl. It prevents contagious diseases and protects people from evil spirits. It is an excellent tonic for healthy people.

Rinchen Ratna bsam-phel
Precious Wish Fulfilling Jewel

This pill is an antidote, for which the recipe comes from the 13th century. It contains precious Ngochu Tsothel, which is produced from detoxified mercury, sulphate and 16 other metals and minerals. There are 16 further constituents, including purified gold, silver, copper, lead and magnetic ironstone, precious stones such as coral, turquoise, pearls, lapis lazuli and the rare Tibetan stone *zi*, as well as clove, bamboo-manna, nutmeg and the fruits of the myrobalans *Terminalia chebula Retz.*, *Terminalia belerica Roxb.* and *Emblica officinalis L.*

The Wish Fulfilling Jewel pill counteracts food poisoning, toxic conditions arising from poisonous plants, insect and animal poisons, chemical toxins and sunburn. It is beneficial for stroke and paralytic fits, for trembling and loss of sensation, dislocated and paralysed limbs as well as in mental illnesses. It is prescribed when there is incontinence from nerve damage, as well as difficulty opening or closing the eyelids. The pill cures deafness, olfactory disorders, loss of body sensation and uncontrolled sputum flow.

It is used to treat high blood pressure, heart disease, tuberculosis and the first stages of cancer. In an advanced stage of cancer it eases pain; and it heals sudden illnesses caused by spirits. When patients take this pill it is as though they are given it directly by the Medicine Buddha. It should be taken on astrologically favourable days, but in an emergency it can be taken immediately.

Rinchen tsha-byor chen-mo
The Great Precious Hot Compound

This pill includes, among other things, detoxified mercury, gold, silver, brass and iron, as well as plants like *Zingiber officinale* (ginger), and shell-ash.

Rinchen tsha-byor chen-mo is used for both cold and hot diseases. It heals *rlung*, *mkhrispa* and *badkan* illnesses, such as headaches, chest infections, limb pains, suppurating wounds, stomach ulcers, gout, arthritis, leprosy, malignant tumours, nervous disorders and oedema.

The evening before taking this 'yellow' precious pill, it should be placed in some beer or wine. The next morning the whole mixture is stirred and drunk, followed by a glass of warm, boiled water.

Rinchen Byur-dmar 25
Precious Coral 25

As the name suggests, this pill contains 25 ingredients – including purified precious stones, coral, pearl, mother-of-pearl and lapis lazuli, as well as saffron, nutmeg, *Crocus sativus L.*, *Saxifraga pasumensis marg.*, and *Terminaloia chebula Retz.*

It is prescribed for headaches, brain afflictions, fainting, fever caused by poisonous substances, neuritis and chronic diseases. This pill can prevent nervous disorders and also counteracts stiffness and paralysis originating in the nervous system.

Emetics, laxatives and inhalations

Emetics and laxatives, as well as enemas, are classified as expelling or purgative

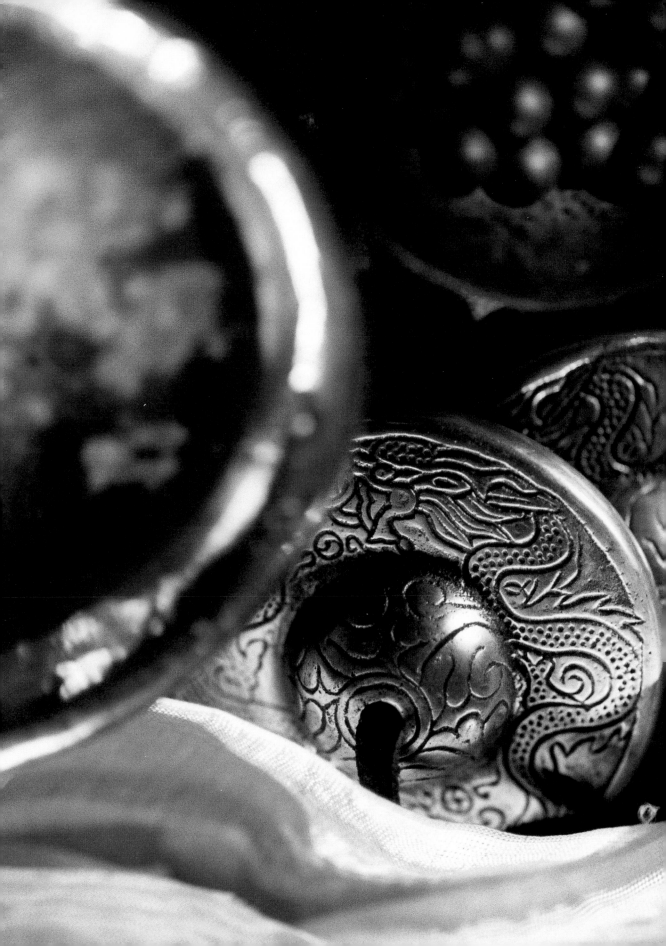

medicines. Laxative cures make use of substances such as castor-oil seeds, cassia pods, various types of nut and rhubarb, and larkspur. Emetics and laxatives are meant to expel excess body fluid and thus free the organism from toxins and deposits. In ancient medical texts, 133 different medicines are suggested for these purposes, but only a few of them are still used today. In general, emetics and laxatives, as well as the inhalation medicines belonging to this group, are seldom prescribed, and then only as a complementary therapy alongside pills.

Laxatives are prescribed for hepatitis, emetics for *badkan* disorders, and inhalations or nose drops for such complaints as headache and earache. Enemas are used for *rlung* illnesses, and inhalations for respiratory tract disorders.

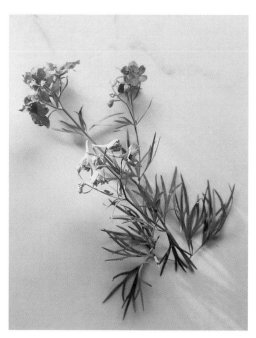

Larkspur is used in laxative cures

Moxibustion

Moxibustion or moxatherapy, together with cupping, is one of the most frequently used external therapies in Tibetan medicine. The moxa herb, dried artemisia (or mugwort), is burned in one of three variations of this therapy:
• The moxa cone is burned directly on the skin
• The moxa cone is burned on an acupuncture needle inserted at particular places in the body
• The moxa cone is burned on a 7cm-long golden needle, about as thick as a knitting needle, which is inserted at certain places in the body. This so-called 'golden moxa' is used specifically for severe cases.
Some types of moxibustion treatment are less painful than others, but it is never entirely painless. This is one of the reasons why it is seldom used for Western patients.

Before treatment begins, the doctor prepares the moxa herb by carefully forming it into small cones by hand. The herb can be burned at different acupuncture points, but the most commonly used is the temple point on the small fontanel (*see page 123*). The selected area is first disinfected either with garlic or (as in Tibetan Medical and Astrological Institute) with an antibiotic cream.

In the first variation the doctor places the moxa cone directly on the skin and allows it to burn up altogether. Eventually the skin glows with heat. Burned scales of skin are rubbed off – usually leaving scars. When the moxa is burned on an acupuncture needle or golden needle, the

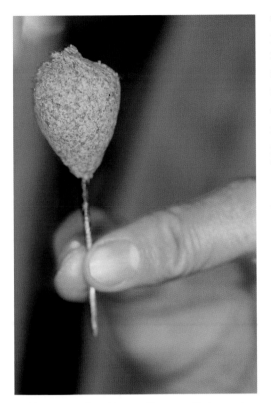

Golden moxa: the golden needle is usually inserted in the vertex acupuncture point. While the moxa cone twisted from artemisia herb burns down, the doctor and patient recite mantras.

as paralysis and brain haemorrhage. In principle it is meant to cause an increase in both white and red blood corpuscles, and thus have a favourable influence on the course of every illness. Yet it is most often applied where body and spirit meet, in the great realm of psychosomatic and psychovegetative disorders, which in the Tibetan system fall into the category of *rlung* illnesses. Moxibustion is even used for cancer, in which case it is applied to a point below the breastbone.

Rituals

There are powerful rituals accompanying moxibustion. While the moxa herb burns, all those present in the room murmur the mantra of the Medicine Buddha: *om namo bagawate bekandsa guru benurja praba radsaja tatagataia arhate samjak sambuddhaja tejata om bekandsa maha bekandsa radsa samogate soha.*

This rhythmic sequence and repetition of sacred syllables is intended to harmonize the patient's disturbed energy patterns. In this way, the ritual addresses the subtle energy body (*see page 53*). The doctor visualizes the Medicine Buddha during this procedure, and as he recites his breath transfers divine power to the patient.

Patients who are to receive moxibustion treatment are summoned to attend on very specific days. These are known as 'heat-treatment days', and are also used for sweat cures, steam therapies and treatments with hot stones or warm sand. It is forbidden to give these treatments on Tuesday, Saturday and Sunday, as these

needle is first inserted into the appropriate acupuncture point, and then the herb is lit.

Moxibustion has an extremely broad range of applications. It not only works at the physical level of the three energies but also on more rarefied processes; and it even addresses the metaphysical level. Thus moxibustion is the favoured healing method for mental illnesses, psychoses and epilepsy, as well as for possession by spirits and demons. Among physical disorders, it is used in severe illnesses such

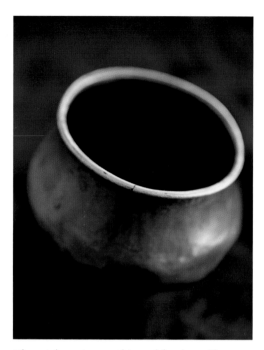

The metal cupping vessel is used for rlung *illnesses.*

days have the same fire nature as the therapy itself.

The first 10 days of the Tibetan month are unfavourable for treating the upper region of the body, the middle 10 days for the middle body and the last 10 days of the month for the lower body.

Cupping

Cupping is part of a Tibetan doctor's daily practice. First the doctor lights a piece of paper (or sometimes a piece of artemisia) and throws it into a round metal cup. This is immediately applied to the patient's body, and the vacuum created makes the cupping vessel suck fast to the skin, where it remains for between 5 and 20 minutes.

When it is removed, the skin underneath will be red and raised. According to Tibetan medicine, toxins collect here. In order to intensify the effect, the doctor will sometimes slit open the area with a fine knife to allow the 'bad blood' to flow off.

Cupping is chiefly performed on the back, at shoulder-blade level, and along the spine. Cupping is commonly prescribed, with or without bloodletting, to treat pain or tension in the neck, shoulders and back, where they are physical signs of *rlung* disorders. Cupping is also an effective treatment for circulatory problems, injuries, bruising and inflammations.

Bloodletting

There are 77 sites in the body where bloodletting is practised. The doctor chooses the site that is related to the organ he is trying to heal. He makes a small slit with a fine knife or stiletto, similar to the way we take blood samples from the fingertip. The tip of the nose and forehead are appropriate for an eye disorder, described by Tibetan doctors as a 'moist accumulation illness'. For headaches a little blood may be taken from the patient's finger and reintroduced through the nostrils. Blood is taken above all in the case of fever and other hot illnesses, though this method is never used for Western patients.

Cauterization

While moxibustion, cupping and bleeding are commonly used by Western naturopaths, cauterization is relatively unknown here. The cauterizing rod is a gold- or copper-pointed metal rod about 20cm long, of up to 1cm in diameter. In surgeries with electricity the cauterizing rod is simply heated on a stove; otherwise it is placed on red-hot coals. The glowing rod is applied to the same sites as for cupping, and the illnesses treated are the same.

Acupuncture with a golden needle

Tibetan acupuncture originally derives from Chinese medicine, but has been further developed and modified. In contrast to Chinese practice, it is prescribed very sparingly and is usually limited to a single, though fairly painful, prick with the golden needle, as described above in the section on moxibustion. The small fontanel at the back of the head, a point to one side of the spine, and over the breastbone, are preferred acupuncture points. This 'golden needle therapy' is used to treat circulatory and brain disorders, mental illness, epilepsy and stroke. The doctor will observe the rules relating to hours, days and seasons in which certain points may not be used, or which are astrologically unfavourable for the patient. As in moxibustion, mantras are recited during golden needle treatment.

Religious cures and rites

Religious cures are the preserve of high-ranking lamas. They address the subtle 'double' body or subtle energy body, as it is described in the *Kalachakra Tantra*, for this is affected when the body falls sick. It is like an interrupted life-force, which is of an unquantifiable and intangible nature. At the point when Western doctors would send their patient to a psychologist because of emotional and mental blockages, or for depression and anxiety, Tibetan medicine turns to the teaching of the subtle double body.

This 'body' can only be perceived during meditation. Spiritual practices help to harmonize it again.

Spiritual cures include 'living the dharma' (following the lifestyle teachings of Buddhism) and reciting mantras; and also the warming Tum-mo yoga meditation, the laying-on of hands, and chakra and colour therapy. Some lamas will use physical deprivation, such as fasting, or prescribe pilgrimages and ritual walks round holy sites (such as Kailash Mountain, or Manasarovar Lake).

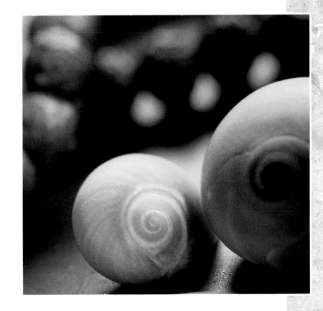

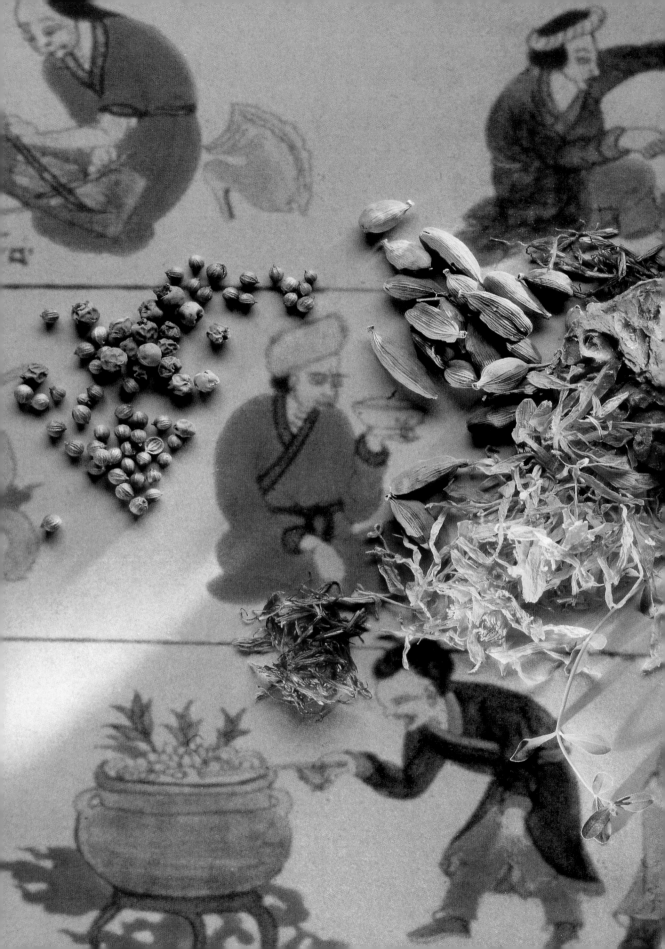

Practical
Applications

3

HEALING PLANTS

The range of herbal remedies used in Tibetan medicine has changed over the centuries. Bon shamans gathered their medicinal herbs exclusively in the Himalayas, but as early as the 4th century AD doctors came from India at the invitation of King Lhathothori Nyentsan, and brought with them the first foreign plants.

Doctors and botanists often find it difficult to identify all the plants referred to in ancient Tibetan medical texts. Errors began to creep in when texts were translated from Sanskrit or Chinese; and some of the plants mentioned in ancient scripts have become extinct. Sometimes lowland plants that were hard to procure were replaced with nearer-to-hand substitutes, which then came to be called by the names of their lowland counterparts. This was further complicated by the effects of recent events in Tibet's history: only a few of the older generation of Tibetan doctors, who still had extensive knowledge of the herbal materia medica, survived the Chinese invasion. But efforts have been made to rediscover ancient knowledge. As well as Tibetan doctors and scholars, a team of scientists at Vienna University have been researching Tibetan plants.

Medicines as compounds

Westerners frequently fall into the trap of trying to ascribe a very specific application to each Tibetan plant. However, Tibetan teachings on medicine manufacture and prescription are based on quite different principles. Although general applications are ascribed to single remedies in medicine texts, Tibetan doctors would never prescribe a single plant. Some of the individual substances used are even regarded as 'toxic' on their own – that is, they create imbalance in the organism.

Tibetan herbal remedies are all compounds. There can be up to a hundred different substances in a single medicine. The formulae are composed of three groups of drugs: main drugs, which have a balancing or restoring effect on disturbed bodily systems; subsidiary drugs, which support and direct the effects of the main drugs; and a third group which protects the body from any harmful side-effects.

The composition of Tibetan prescriptions depends on a complex system of classification, which we can only describe here in simplified form. Drugs are primarily categorized according to whether they restore equilibrium for hot or cold illnesses, or whether they are neutral in this regard. This information is derived from the taste spheres (*ro*), the active forces (*nuspa*), the taste spheres after digestion (*zuryes*) and the qualities (*yontan*). Further criteria for determining a plant's application include its scent, colour and form.

Previous pages – A section of the medicine thangka *number 22, representing Tibetan nutritional lore. Strewn over it are healing plants and spices, including saffron, marigold, lotus seeds, cardamom, pepper, nutmeg blossom and sandalwood.*
Opposite – Medicine thangka *number 1: Buddha Shakyamuni proclaims the 'knowledge of healing'.*

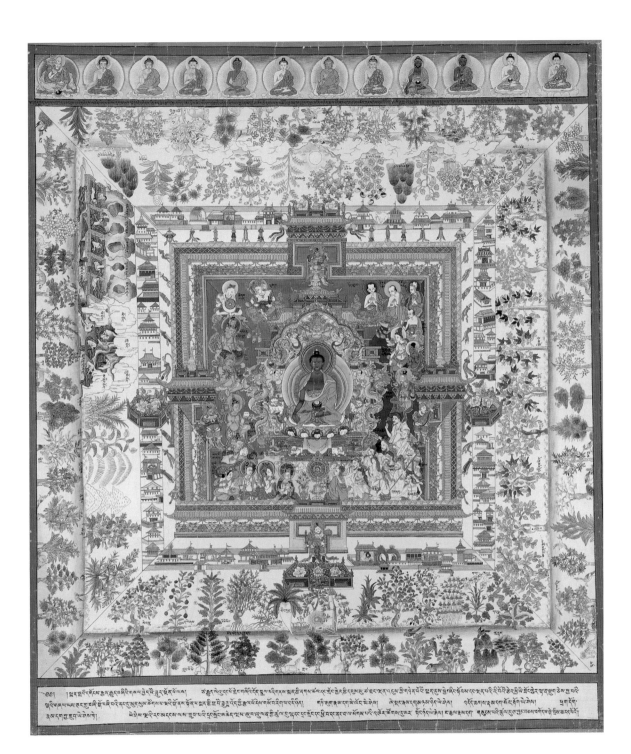

According to Buddhists, the whole of Tibetan medical knowledge can be traced back to the Buddha Shakyamuni. The Medicine Buddha also explained herbal lore, together with the classification of plants according to whether they have a cooling or warming active force. This is described in the introduction to the *Root Tantra* in the *rGyudbzh*, the basic book of medical teachings, which in the 17th century was interpreted through the *Blue Beryl (see page 18)*. At the time, artists painted the famous 79 medical scroll paintings on silk. The first of these *thangkas* represents the proclamation of Tibetan medicine. Here follows a literal translation from the *rGyudbzhi* (in italics) and the *Blue Beryl* (names of the plants):

The perfect teacher, the Medicine Buddha, proclaims knowledge of healing in a perfect town surrounded by four mountains, upon which good medicinal plants grow.

In the south rises 'bigshyed (big-tsche) mountain, 'the cutting one', which possesses the power of the sun. There one can find remedies such as pomegranate, black pepper, long pepper, white Cayenne pepper (tsitraka) etc., which heal illnesses of a cold nature. The plants of its forests are of sharp, sour and salty taste; their active forces are warming and sharp. The medicinal roots, stems, branches, leaves, flowers and fruit are fragrant, attractive and lovely to behold, and wherever their scent spreads no cold illness will appear.

The plants depicted provide the medicinal ingredients: pomegranate, black pepper, long pepper, Cayenne pepper (*tsitraka*), Asafoetida, Sumac, cinnamon, cassia bark, pine trunk, forest vine, rhododendron, ginger, buttercup and Bonducella fruit.

In the north rises the mountain gangstchen (kangtschen), 'the snow-rich', which possesses the power of the moon. There can be found remedies such as sandalwood, camphor, aloeswood, nim etc., which cure illnesses of a hot or warm nature. In its forests grow plants which bring forth medicines of bitter, sweet and astringent taste, and with cool, dull active forces. The medicinal roots, stems, branches, leaves, flowers and fruit are fragrant, attractive and lovely to behold, and wherever their scent spreads no hot illness will appear.

The plants depicted provide the medicinal ingredients: white sandalwood, camphor, aloeswood, nim, tarantula, liquorice, coleus leaves, monkshood, red sandalwood, golden saxifrage, kapok and grapevine.

In the East rises the mountain sposngadldan (poenyeden), 'the aromatic one', which possesses the power of sun and moon equally. Here grows a forest of myrobalan trees. All parts of this tree are used as medicine: the roots (bone diseases), the trunk (muscular diseases), the twigs (diseases of the blood vessels and ligaments), the bark (skin diseases), the leaves (diseases of the cavity organs), the flowers (diseases of the sense organs), and the fruits named arura, the myrobalan fruits (diseases of the heart and other major organs). In their topmost branches ripen the five varieties of myrobalan, which combine the six taste spheres, the eight active forces, the three taste spheres after digestion, and the sixteen qualities. And wherever these fragrant, attractive and agreeable medicines appear, none of the four hundred and four illnesses arise.

Depicted are: the 'vanquishing', the 'fearless', the 'nectar-', the 'enriching', the 'dry', the 'small black', the 'golden' and the 'beak-shaped' myrobalan.

In the West rises the mountain Malaya, also possessing the power of sun and moon. On this mountain grow six excellent remedies.

The five varieties of limestone, the five varieties of pure bitumen, the five varieties of healing spring and five varieties of thermal spring heal all illnesses.

The plants depicted provide the following medicinal ingredients: nutmeg, clove, bamboo concretion, saffron, small cardamom and great cardamom.

PLANT DESCRIPTIONS

The plants described here all have different applications in Tibetan medicine, which are listed below along with their classifications in the *rGyudbzhi* and the *Blue Beryl*. It is important that you don't

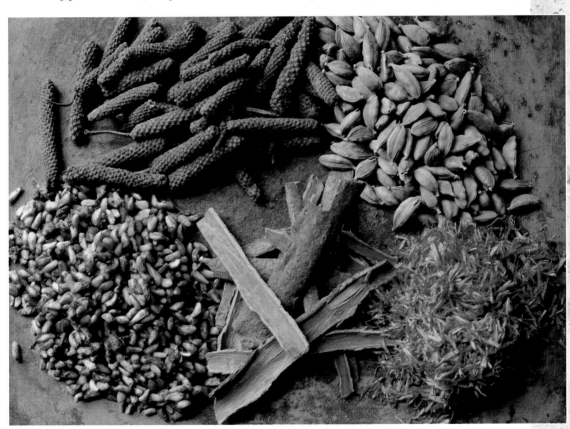

Ingredients of a herbal formula called 'Men-Chik': pomegranate seeds, long pepper, small cardamom, safflower and cinnamon.

attempt to treat yourself based on these descriptions. Before taking Tibetan medicine, it is advisable to obtain an accurate diagnosis from a Tibetan doctor. Tibetan herbal medicines tend to work in combinations rather than as individual remedies, and it requires expertise to understand how to combine separate remedies to achieve a subtly graded, specific result, with minimum side-effects. The plant descriptions here give an idea of the highly developed system underlying the production of remedies. Pharmacology is one of the most difficult and complex areas of Tibetan medicine, and aspiring pharmacologists must complete a further study of several years in addition to their medical studies. All herb pills, not just the 'precious pills', are small works of art – the quintessence of thousands of years of meditative research, and they deserve enormous respect.

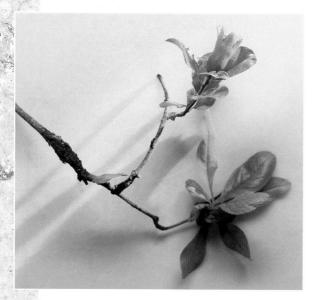

Pomegranate

The South Mountain
Medicines for cold illnesses

Pomegranate

Punica granatum L.; *Punicaceae*

The pomegranate tree is indigenous to a wide area stretching from the Himalayas across to the Mediterranean. This deciduous tree, with its blood-red or sometimes yellow blossoms, is very attractive, but nowadays is chiefly cultivated for its fruit, in tropical and subtropical regions of the globe. The blossoms ripen into apple-sized fruits enclosed in their red-yellow sepals. In the fruit's interior are its pea-sized seeds. The outer part of the seed becomes red and fleshy when ripe. These seed-fruits are delicious to eat: they are sucked or chewed and the seeds themselves are often spat out. Grenadine syrup is made from pomegranate juice and in India the roots, bark, blossoms, fruit and seeds are used for medicinal purposes.

TIBETAN NAME AND CHARACTERIZATION

The pomegranate is called *se'bru* (sendu). The seeds are used as a medicine. The juicy seed-fruit is simply allowed to dry over the actual seeds, which are then ground to a powder. This drug is ascribed the taste of sour and sweet, as well as the active force of oily. In medical texts *se'bru* is often given as the prime example of a sour drug. Among other things *se'bru* has an excellent warming effect on digestion. There are numerous formulae containing *se'bru* as a main component. Depending on the other ingredients added, the warming effect of the drug can be directed to different organs, for instance the stomach, intestine or kidneys.

Black pepper

Piper nigrum L.; Piperaceae

Black pepper is obtained from a climbing plant that probably originated in southern India. Nowadays this is used as a spice throughout the world, and cultivated in the tropics. This perennial plant can reach a height of up to 15 metres with the aid of its clinging roots, similar to ivy. From the leaf-nodes grow spikes with tiny blossoms, which ripen into red, berry-like fruit. To obtain black pepper the fruits are harvested as they start to turn red, and left to dry in the sun or by a fire. White pepper, on the other hand, is obtained from fully ripe fruit, by first removing the fruit-flesh and then drying the seeds.

TIBETAN NAME AND CHARACTERIZATION

Black pepper is called *nalesham* (na-le-sham) in Tibetan. It is counted among the medicines of sharp taste, and with sharp, hot and harsh active forces, which counteract *badkan* disorders and increase *mkhrispa*. It is this property of black pepper that, among other things, helps to stimulate the digestion.

Long pepper

Piper longum L.; Piperaceae

This type of pepper is indigenous to all the evergreen subtropical forests of Asia and the eastern Himalayas. The long pepper usually comes from northern India, but is also cultivated in southern India and can be bought in specialist shops in the UK. This is a perennial climbing plant which

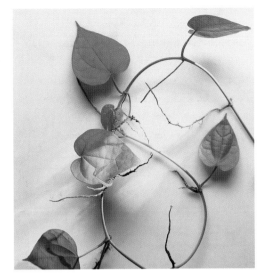

Black pepper

resembles black pepper, but is more delicate in form. The yellow blossoms develop into red, berry-type fruit, but these are deeply embedded in the fleshy spike, forming a kind of cone. The whole dried spikes are used, together with their ripe fruit. In India the roots of this plant are also used for medicinal purposes.

TIBETAN NAME AND CHARACTERIZATION

Long pepper is called *pipiling* (pi-pi-ling) in Tibetan. Once dried it has a sharp taste with a sweet taste after digestion. It is one of the medicines that can cure cold and specially *badkan* illnesses; but in contrast to black pepper it does not increase the *mkhrispa* bodily energy. Long pepper is prescribed as an expectorant, and is effective for coughs.

Ginger

Zingiber officinale Rosc.; Zingiberaceae

The ginger plant comes from southern Asia, but nowadays it can only be found growing wild in some parts of India. It is cultivated in southern China, India, Japan, the West Indies, Central America and Africa. Dried ginger reached Europe in ancient times, and was used there for culinary purposes. In the regions where it is cultivated, fresh ginger is often used as a digestion-enhancing additive to foods. The ginger plant is a slender perennial that reproduces through underground rhizome division. In the spring, a 1-metre-long leaf shoot bearing smooth, lancet-like leaves grows from the rhizome. The blossom-bearing organs grow directly from the rhizome, and bear at their topmost point a cylindrical spike with a yellow-green blossom. In contrast to the perennial rhizome, the parts above ground die back each year. After harvesting, the fleshy, starch-rich rhizomes are thrown into boiling water and afterwards dried.

TIBETAN NAME AND CHARACTERIZATION

Ginger has various different Tibetan names. Dried 'medicinal' ginger that is processed into medicine is called *smangsa* (men-ga). Fresher ginger, which is still moist, is called *spagsher* (ga-sher). *Sgakya* (gakya), meaning literally 'white ginger', is also the name for fresh ginger. It is not clear whether the wild ginger referred to in the *Blue Beryl* is simply freshly gathered ginger or another type altogether. At any rate, some texts assign wild ginger to the species *Hedychium spicatum*, another member of the ginger family whose rhizomes are used as medicine. To wild (fresh) ginger are ascribed the taste spheres of sweet and sharp, and the active force of hot and oily. In general, ginger is

believed to increase heat in the body, to stimulate appetite and overcome *badkan* disorders. Thus *spagsher* is regarded as a remedy for hangovers.

Cayenne pepper
Capsicum frutescens L.; Solanaceae

This perennial bush, indigenous to south and central America, grows only in the tropics, and produces 1.5- to 3-centimetre-long, shining red, pointed berries, loosely known as 'pods'. The less pungent variety, with slightly larger fruit, from which paprika is obtained – *Capsicum annuum* – was introduced to India soon after the conquest of the New World. From there it was brought to England as early as 1548, and was known to English herbal doctors of that time. We can assume that Cayenne pepper itself soon found its way to India and was cultivated there.

TIBETAN NAME AND CHARACTERIZATION

Cayenne pepper is called *tsitraka* (tsi-tra-ka). Its extremely sharp taste makes it a strongly warming medicine, and it is often known as the 'king of heat'. In some books, however, leadwort (*Plumbago zeylanica*) – a climbing, shrub-like plant indigenous to south-east Asia whose twigs are used medicinally – is given the name *tsitraka* and the title 'king of heat'. What is the solution to this botanical conundrum? In the *rGyudbzhi*, reference is made to *tsitraka* and its warming character, but no description of the plant is provided. It is possible that leadwort was the sole 'king of heat' at the time the *rGyudbzhi* was written, before Cayenne pepper came from the New World to compete with it. In the chapter on materia medica, the medical scroll paintings clearly depict a Cayenne pepper plant as *tsitraka*. But in the 'proclamation' scene (*see page 57*) on the other hand, the upright fruits portrayed more closely resemble the leadwort. Because their taste sphere and active forces are the same, both plants are nowadays used as *tsitraka*.

Asafoetida

Ferula assa-foetida L. and Ferula narthex Boiss.; Umbelliferae

Ferula assa-foetida grows wild in the Punjab, Kashmir, Iran, Afghanistan and Turkestan, and *Ferula narthex* grows in the north-western Himalayas. These perennials, with their umbels of 10 to 20 blossoms each, belong to the same family as cow-parsley. They grow to a height of 1.8 to 33 metres, and have a huge, fleshy, carrot-like root with one or two forks. The roots of four- to five-year-old plants are exposed shortly before the plant blossoms, and the parts of the plant above ground are cut off. The exposed surface of root is then covered with twigs and earth. After a few days the milky latex exuded is scraped off. Root slices are repeatedly cut off until no more of this sap appears. It is dried and then sold in flat, round sheets.

TIBETAN NAME AND CHARACTERIZATION

Asafoetida is called *shingkun* (shing-kuen) in Tibetan, and is used for cold illnesses and for deworming. *Shingkun* is the main ingredient of a formula with a digestion-enhancing, anti-flatulence effect. In some regions of India, asafoetida is used as a culinary spice.

Cinnamon

Cinnamomum verum J.S.Presl and Cinnamomum aromaticum Nees; Lauraceae

Cinnamon is derived from two different trees: the cinnamon tree that grows wild in Sri Lanka (*Cinnamomum verum*), and is cultivated in India, Sri Lanka, Indonesia, the West Indies and Brazil; and the cinnamon cassia, which is indigenous to the Indian sub-continent and Kwangsi in China (*Cinnamomum aromaticum*).

Wild, evergreen cinnamon trees grow up to 20 metres high, but when they are cultivated they are usually kept bush-like, in the same way as the basket willow tree is cultivated. The bark of their shoots is used as both spice and medicine. Two-year-old plants are cut down and their bark is peeled. The pieces of bark are left to ferment overnight, and on the following day the outer bark layers are scraped off, leaving the inner layers which contain the highest concentration of cinnamon. These pieces of bark are dried first in the shade then in sunlight. In the case of cinnamon cassia, the thicker pieces of bark are used, without scraping.

TIBETAN NAME AND CHARACTERIZATION

The Tibetan name for cinnamon is *shingtsa* (shing-tsa). Cinnamon has the taste spheres of sharp, sweet, astringent and salty. According to the *Blue Beryl*, both kinds of cinnamon can be used medicinally. The one with the thinner bark has a warmer active force than the one with thicker bark. Cinnamon counteracts cold illnesses of the stomach and liver, as well as providing a good defence against cold *rlung* and *badkan* disorders.

The North Mountain
Medicines for hot illnesses

White sandalwood
Santalum album L.; *Santalaceae*

This tree is found from the Indian peninsula to Malaysia. It grows best in dry regions at an altitude of up to 1,200 metres. In India there are great plantations of sandalwood trees, and the sandalwood industry is a state monopoly. This evergreen tree, which flowers all year round, has lancet-oval leaves up to 6 centimetres long, and it grows as high as 18 metres. It leads a semi-parasitic existence: a few months after germinating, its roots insinuate themselves into the roots of annual plants and small bushes. Later it feeds off the roots of trees. For this reason, sandalwood plantations should always have suitable host plants. The tree grows very slowly and is often only felled after 50 to 60 years. Distillation of the woody parts of the tree produces different qualities of oil, which are then used either in the cosmetics industry, for making perfume, or to produce homeopathic medicine. In India, incense sticks are made from the heart-wood that remains once the bark and sapwood have been removed. Until antibiotics were discovered, Western doctors used sandalwood oil as an antimicrobial remedy in urinary tract infections. However, the oil had to be administered in a stomach acid-resistant capsule because of the danger of stomach irritation. One of the advantages of Tibetan remedies is that they always include substances to protect other organs.

TIBETAN NAME AND CHARACTERIZATION

In Tibetan medicine, both wood and oil are used. The sandalwood tree is called *tsandan dkarpo* (tsen-den kar-po) in Tibetan. The taste of the substance is astringent, the active force cooling. White sandalwood is the chief component of several remedies prescribed for inflammations and infections.

Camphor
Cinnamomum camphora (L.) J.S. Presl.; *Lauracaea*

The camphor tree is indigenous to the hardwood forests of China, Taiwan and southern Japan, and from there it has been introduced to all continents. It is chiefly cultivated in China, Japan, Taiwan, the USA and the former Soviet Union. This evergreen tree of the laurel family can grow up to 40 metres high and develops an enormous girth. Longish, oval leaves grow from its knotty branches. Depending on its purity, camphor is an amorphous or crystalline powder that is obtained from the tree's wood and leaves by water distillation and subsequent sublimation. During distillation, camphor oil is also exuded, which is used in aromatherapy and for industrial purposes. Camphor is a very ancient remedy particularly valued by the Arabs. According to the Qu'ran, the drink of the blessed was spiced with camphor. Arabic camphor comes from another tree, *Dryobalanops aromatica*, in which the camphor is distilled within the trunk of the tree itself, through sublimation. This camphor was far more expensive than the laurel-camphor common today. *Dryobalanops camphor* was also known in Central Europe in the Middle Ages, and was displaced by the cheaper laurel camphor in the 16th century. Hildegard of Bingen noted that it was good for fever, and restored strength to sick people. It hinders inflammation and works as an analeptic, stimulating the respiratory and circulatory systems.

TIBETAN NAME AND CHARACTERIZATION

In Tibet camphor is called *gabur*. There are three types and qualities, depending on the tree from which it is extracted: white, yellow and wrinkled, and one which appears in long, shining yellow pieces. *Gabur* has the taste spheres bitter, sharp and astringent, and the active force cooling. It is included in formulae against all types of fever (in Tibetan medicine, six different kinds of fever are described, which have many other characteristics aside from a raised temperature).

Nim tree

Azadirachta indica A. Juss.; *Meliaceae*

The nim tree is indigenous to India, Burma, Sri Lanka and the Malayan archipelago, and is also cultivated outside this region. It is the holy tree of the Hindus and can be admired in many gardens. The Indians use all parts of this imposing, evergreen 'miracle tree', which grows as high as 20 metres but only has scant foliage. From it they produce fertilizer, insecticides, dyes, wax, lubricants, soap and a great many other products.

TIBETAN NAME AND CHARACTERIZATION

In Tibet it is mainly the twigs and leaves of the *nimpa*, as it is called, that are used medicinally. The taste of the drug is very

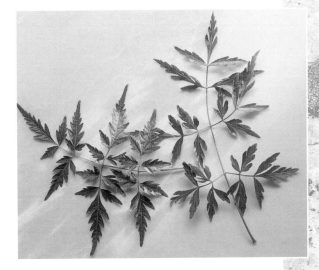

Nim tree

bitter. It is traditionally prescribed for hot illnesses, loss of appetite, bad breath and certain skin diseases.

Red sandalwood

Pterocarpus santalinus L.; *Leguminosae*

This tree grows up to 7.5 metres tall and is indigenous to southern India, but since it is a protected species it is also cultivated. It is a very pretty deciduous tree with broad elliptical leaves and bunches of yellow blossom. A dark brown bark encloses the lighter sapwood. In the interior lies the extremely hard and dark purple heartwood. Once the sapwood is removed, this heartwood is ground to powder and used for medicinal purposes. The heartwood was formerly also used for dyeing wool. The numbers of red sandalwood have greatly declined, because of the general destruction of tropical forests as well as its use as a dye. Its medicinal use in India as a remedy for disorders of the stomach and intestinal tract, a diuretic, astringent and 'blood purifying medicine', and for coughing, has probably not had much influence on its decline.

TIBETAN NAME AND CHARACTERIZATION

The tree producing red sandalwood is called tsandan *dmarpo* (tsen-den mar-po) in Tibetan. It has an astringent taste, and is one of the remedies that ease hot illnesses.

Liquorice

Glycyrrhiza glabra L.; Leguminosae

The liquorice plant is indigenous to the Mediterranean, Asia Minor, Iran and Syria, but has spread as far as China; nowadays it is cultivated in the Mediterranean, Russia and India (the lower Himalayas and the Punjab). In the Middle Ages it was also grown in Central Europe. In Mongolia the variety *Glycyrrhiza uralensis Fisch.* is cultivated, which is used in the Tibetan medicine of Buryat. This perennial reproduces via underground runners and has a woody, yellow root. Bunches of violet or yellow-white papilionaceous flowers grow from the leaf nodes of the pinnate leaves. The roots are used for both medical and culinary purposes. In the West, the thickened sap of the roots produces the much-loved liquorice sweet. For medical purposes the roots are processed into powder or extracts.

TIBETAN NAME AND CHARACTERIZATION

In Tibetan medicine, the roots of the *shinmngar* (shing-gar), as it is called, are used. The medicine has a sweet taste and is included as a component in remedies to counteract lung diseases. Western herbal medicine also recommends liquorice as an expectorant for colds, bronchial catarrh, hoarseness and coughs.

The East Mountain
Medicines from the myrobalan tree

Chebula myrobalan

Terminalia chebula (Gaertn.)n Retz.; Combretaceae

This medium-sized, broad-leaved tree grows in deciduous woods on dry slopes, in many Asiatic regions including Malaysia and northern India. The leaves are alternate, and ovoid or elliptic. There are distinctive hanging fruits, 2 to 4 centimetres in length, which are black, orange–brown or yellow and usually elliptical or ovoid in shape.

TIBETAN NAME AND CHARACTERIZATION

The *arura* (a-ru-ra) fruits, the myrobalans, have a central place in Tibetan medicine. Their importance is symbolized in pictures of the Buddha Shakyamuni, who as master of medicines always offers myrobalan fruits or branches. In ancient medical texts several different varieties of myrobalans are distinguished: 'vanquishing', 'fearless', 'nectar', 'enriching', 'dry', 'small black', 'golden' and 'beak-shaped'.

According to the *rGyudbzhi*, the 'vanquishing myrobalan' symbolized the perfect remedy. It combined all six taste spheres, the eight active forces, the three taste spheres after digestion, and the sixteen qualities; and was able to cure all illnesses arising from *rlung*, *mkhrispa* and *badkan* disorders, as well as all hot and cold illnesses. According to tradition, this type of myrobalan only grows when a Medicine Buddha appears on Earth. It is probably a symbol of our human longing for such a medicine. The 'golden myrobalan' fruit is closest to this in appearance, since it is neck-shaped like the 'vanquishing' one. The varieties growing today only combine five of the taste spheres (salty is missing), and are used for illnesses that arise from *rlung*, *mkhrispa* and *badkan* disorders.

The 'fearless' myrobalan fruit is black and longish and is recommended for eye complaints. The 'nectar' myrobalan is yellow, has thick flesh and helps emaciated people to put on weight. The 'enriching' myrobalan has the shape of a vase and is recommended for wounds. The 'dry' myrobalan fruit is thin and very wrinkled. It cures *mkhrispa* disorders in children. The 'beak-shaped' myrobalan is long and pointed, and is regarded as a laxative. The 'small black' myrobalan has no seeds, and its medicinal properties are similar to the 'nectar' myrobalan. Remember, though, that a single substance is never prescribed on its own. These classifications serve doctors as an aid to finding the most suitable type of fruit to include in compound formulae. In general the myrobalans are considered to aid digestion, and have a life-enhancing, nourishing and strengthening effect on the body. They form part of many prescriptions as a supporting ingredient.

Bellirica myrobalan
Terminalia bellirica (Gaertn.) Roxb.; Combretaceae

The bellirica myrobalan tree can be found in the same regions as the chebula myrobalan. This deciduous tree with thick, brown-grey bark, grows to a height of 20 to 30 metres. Its foliage consists of broad,

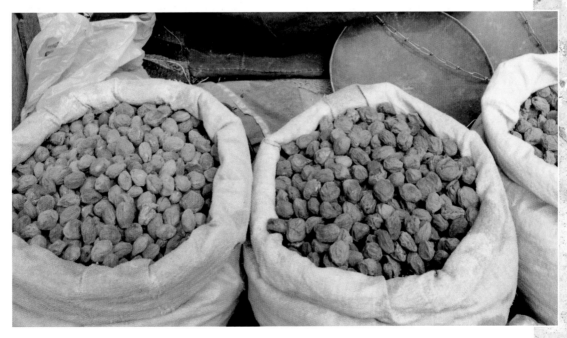

Bellirica myrobalan fruits

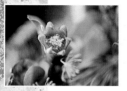

elliptical leaves which chiefly sprout from the ends of the twigs. The blossoms are yellow-green with an unpleasant odour, and they produce pentagonal, fig-shaped fruits.

TIBETAN NAME AND CHARACTERIZATION
The fruits of this tree are called *barura*, and the medicine's active force is hot. There are various qualities of barura, and the yellow fruits are considered to be the best. All types are used against *badkan* and *mkhrispa* illnesses, for lymph diseases, and in balancing *rlung* disorders.

Emblica myrobalan

Emblica officinalis Gaertn.; Euphorbiacaea

This tree is indigenous to India and the deciduous forests of the Himalayas. It is also cultivated in the lowlands.

The plant belongs to the spurge family, and is therefore not related to the other myrobalan species. There are no trees of this species in central Europe, so the appearance of this 8- to 18-metre deciduous tree is unfamiliar to us. Close ranks of small, simple leaves sprout from the delicate branches and male and female flowers bloom on the lower twigs. Round, fleshy, pale-yellow fruits with six notches develop from the female flowers.

TIBETAN NAME AND CHARACTERIZATION
These *skyurura* (kyu-ru-ra) fruit are used for medicinal purposes. Their taste is described as sour, their active force as cool. This medicine balances disorders of the three bodily energies *rlung*, *mkhrispa* and *badkan*, and helps cure blood diseases.

Seven excellent medicines

Nutmeg

Myristica fragrans Houtt.; Myristiceae

The nutmeg tree is an evergreen plant with two forms, male and female. Although it can grow as high as 20 metres, it is usually kept small in cultivation. The female plants form one to three blossoms in the leaf nodes, which, once pollinated, develop into peach-type fruits. The seed – wrongly called a 'nut' – in each fruit is enclosed in a bright red shell. Once dried, this is sold as nutmeg mace. The seeds are dried and then cracked open to get the kernels, which are used for various purposes. Rich nutmeg oil can be obtained by hot pressing.

TIBETAN NAME AND CHARACTERIZATION
In Tibetan medicine the fruits and the oil are used. The fruits are processed into powder for pills, while the oil is used in massage. Nutmeg is called *dzati* (zati) in Tibetan. The tree itself is called *shingsnama* (shing-na-ma). Its taste is sharp, the active force oily. Among other things, *dzati* counteracts *rlung* disorders and stimulates digestion. *Dzati* is also the name given to a formula that contains 20 ingredients and counteracts *rlung* disorders. This remedy also has a beneficial effect on the nervous system, combating insomnia, irritability and anxiety.

Clove

Syzygium aromaticum (L.) Merr. et Perry; Myrtaceae

The clove tree, indigenous to the Moluccas, is now cultivated in Indonesia,

Sri Lanka, southern India, Madagascar, Zanzibar, on islands of the Indian Ocean, and in the American tropics. It is a tropical evergreen tree growing from 10 to 12 metres high, and from its sixth year of growth onwards produces umbels at the ends of its branches, with numerous flowers. The flower buds are plucked before they open, for it is then that they contain most oil. After harvesting they are dried in the sun or by a fire. Numerous oil glands secrete essential oils, consisting of 70 to 90 per cent eugenol. Eugenol has strongly antiseptic and pain-relieving properties, and is also used in Western dentistry practice.

TIBETAN NAME AND CHARACTERIZATION

The Tibetan name for this medicine is *lishi*. According to the *rGyudbzhi* it is effective against diseases of the respiratory system, cold *rlung* illnesses and hoarseness. Clove is the chief one of six ingredients in a popular remedy for hoarseness and respiratory infections.

Bamboo concretion

Bambusa arundinaceae (Retz.) Willd.; Gramineae

This thorny bamboo variety is found all over India at altitudes of 2,100 metres. A bush-type plant, it grows up to 3 metres high. Many closely packed shoots grow from each thick rootstock. The shoots form characteristic nodes every 45 centimetres, from which, in this particular type, thorns also grow.

TIBETAN NAME AND CHARACTERIZATION

In Tibetan medicine, only the bamboo concretion (a substance that collects inside the shoots) is used. In India, this is known as bamboo-manna. The medicine made from it is called *chugang*. True bamboo concretion is yellow-grey when it is harvested from bamboo. Its taste is indefinite or sweet, its active force dull. In the *Blue Beryl* a *chugang* of mineral origin is described, which is white and without taste. Bamboo concretion is used to heal illnesses of the lungs and traumatic fever among other things. There are several formulae in which *chugang* is the main ingredient, two of which are specifically for children.

Saffron

Crocus sativus L.; Iridaceae

The plant from which saffron is obtained comes originally from Asia Minor. It was first cultivated in the distant past, and now it is only known as a cultivated plant. It is grown in Mediterranean countries, Russia and India (Kashmir and Jammu, at altitudes above 1,600 metres), among other places. *Crocus sativus* is a rosette plant growing up to 25 centimetres high, with linear leaves. A purplish-blue flower sprouts from the tuber in October, with an appearance similar to our spring crocus. The dried stigmas of the blossoms are used both for dyeing and medicinal purposes. The 10-centimetre-long style holds three orange-red stigmas which, after arduous harvesting, are dried. To make one kilogram of saffron, 150,000 to 200,000 stigmas are required! It is therefore hardly surprising that this spice is very expensive.

TIBETAN NAME AND CHARACTERIZATION

In Tibetan, saffron is called *khache-gurgum* (kash-gur-gum). In India, Kashmir saffron is still regarded as the best quality. In the *Blue Beryl* a Nepalese *gurgum* is also mentioned, and is said to grow as tall as a man. However this is the safflower (*Carthamus tinctorius*) whose blossoms are used in Tibet as a substitute for the more precious saffron. Apart from these two plants, the flowers of Calendula varieties are also used in Tibet as a saffron substitute. Since today's *gurgum* prescriptions often cite safflower as a chief constituent, the taste and active force of *gurgum* are listed under 'safflower'.

Safflower
Carthamus tinctorius L.; *Compositae*

This plant has been used from very ancient times for dyes and oil. It was probably indigenous to the Orient but it is now cultivated all over the world. Its blossoms provide a red dye, carthamine, which was also produced in European plantations until the discovery of aniline dyes. An oil is pressed from its seeds that is used both for culinary and industrial purposes. The safflower was either cultivated in Tibet, or brought from Nepal and India. This 70- to 130-centimetre high plant, with spiky, toothed leaves, looks rather like a thistle. At the ends of its forked shoots there are yellow-orange compound flowers 3 centimetres long, which are also guarded by thorny sepals. These are harvested in July and August, as soon as the petals turn orange-red, then they are dried in a well-aired, shady place.

TIBETAN NAME AND CHARACTERIZATION
The blossoms are used in Tibetan medicine. As mentioned under saffron (above), safflower is also called *gurgum*. Nepal *gurgum* is safflower, while Kashmir *gurgum* is saffron. *Gurgum* has the taste spheres sweet and bitter, and the active force of cool. It is the chief constituent of a number of formulae prescribed for different ailments: 'fever' illnesses, liver diseases, and for sealing 'channels' – for instance, to stop the flow of blood.

Small cardamom
Elettaria cardamomum (L.) Maton; *Zingiberaceae*

This reed-like perennial is indigenous to the humid mountainous forests of the Malabar coast, and is cultivated in India and Sri Lanka. Cardamom was known to the Greeks and Romans via the Arab world, and was used in Germany in the Middle Ages. Roughly 3-metre-high, sterile leaf shoots, with long, lancet-type leaves, sprout from fleshy rhizomes; and 8 to 12 white flowers blossom at the top of short, pointed flower spikes. The ovaries develop into pods with three compartments, which contain 12 to 24 seeds altogether. Whole pods or ground seeds can be bought.

TIBETAN NAME AND CHARACTERIZATION
Cardamom is called *sugsmel* (sug-mel) in Tibetan, and the seeds are used in medicine. According to the *rGyudbzhi* it cures all cold kidney and *rlung* illnesses. Cardamom is present as a subsidiary constituent in many formulae.

Large cardamom
Amomum subulatum (*sabulatum*) Roxb.; *Zingiberaceae*

The large cardamom is indigenous to the eastern Himalayas, the older brother of the small cardamom. However, it does not get its name from the height of the plant – it only grows to about 1 metre – but from the fruit. Up to 2.5 centimetres in diameter, the fruits are roughly twice as big as those of the small cardamom. The dried seeds from the fruit capsules are also used.

TIBETAN NAME AND CHARACTERIZATION

In Tibetan this plant is called *kakola*. Its taste is sharp, the active force is hot and harsh. *Kakola* helps re-establish the warmth of digestion (*medrod*), which is responsible for the effective processing of food in the human body, and so it counteracts flatulence and a sense of over-fullness. Large cardamom is present as a subsidiary constituent in many formulae.

Further plants

Saussurea
Saussurea costus (Falc.) Lipschitz; Compositae

This plant can be found in the northern Himalayas, in northern India, Kashmir and Jammu, on damp slopes between 2,500 and 4,000 metres. In some parts of these regions and in certain areas of China, this plant is also cultivated. It is a perennial, growing up to 2 metres high, and bears on its single stem a few dark blue to almost black compound flowers of about 3 centimetres in diameter. It forms a strong root up to 60 centimetres long, which is dug up and dried for medicinal use.

TIBETAN NAME AND CHARACTERIZATION

Saussurea costus is one of the plants called *rurta* (ru-ta) in Tibetan. However, its botanical identity is not clear. In ancient medical texts *rurta* is also described as a plant with white blossoms, and with

characteristics that show it is not a saussurea. In Tibetan medicine, the name of one medicine is often ascribed to several different types of plant or varieties of drug. Sometimes different plants serve as substitutes for medicines that are not readily available; and sometimes, too, a subtly different effect is ascribed to these different varieties, which experienced pharmacologists can make use of. *Rurta* has the taste spheres sharp, sweet and bitter. The effect on hot and cold illnesses is neutral, so the medicine can be used in either case.

In the *rGyudbzhi*, *rurta* is counted among the remedies that cure fever arising from a *rlung* disorder. There are several traditional formulae with *rurta* as their chief constituent, which are prescribed in the case of stomach and intestinal complaints. *Rurta* is also widely used as a subsidiary ingredient.

Rhubarb root
Rheum palmatum L.; Polygonaceae

Rhubarb root is indigenous to the mountains of eastern Tibet and north-west China, and grows there in high bush-scrub at the uppermost forest line. The plant is chiefly cultivated in China and in the former Soviet Union. This strong perennial grows up to 1.5 metres high and lives for as long as 20 to 30 years. During the first few years a rosette forms upon the ground, from which a flower shoot rises sometimes more than 2 metres high. The root system is a beet-type growth, which swells after a few years to 10 to 15 centimetres in diameter, and puts out side-roots which

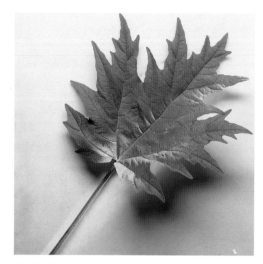

Rhubarb root

colour on the outside is a yellow-green or a yellow-brown.

TIBETAN NAME AND CHARACTERIZATION
In Tibetan medicine the fruit is called *bilba* (bil-va). It has a bitter and astringent taste and an oily active force. This medicine is used in the treatment of diarrhoea and to aid the digestion.

are as thick as an arm. In Western herbal medicine the roots of 3- to 4-year-old plants are used.

TIBETAN NAME AND CHARACTERIZATION
The taste of this plant, known by the name of *lchumrtsa* (tshum-tsa), is sour, sweet and astringent, and the active force is harsh. *Lchumrtsa* has laxative effects, but whereas Western herbalists only use it for this purpose, in Tibetan medicine it is also used in remedies for quite different ailments, such as an upset stomach and acute or chronic disturbance of the three bodily energies.

Coriander
Coriandrum sativum L; *Umbelliferae*

Coriander is an ancient healing plant, mentioned in Egyptian papyri. It comes from the near East and is nowadays cultivated in the Balkans, Russia, Morocco and Europe.

During its first year coriander forms a rosette, from which a 50-centimetre high, forking flower stem then develops. The umbels are composed of white to reddish flowers that ripen into round fruit. These dried and ground fruits are mainly used to spice bread and pastries.

TIBETAN NAME AND CHARACTERIZATION
Excellent medical properties are ascribed to coriander, known as *wusu* in Tibetan. It is used in different ways depending on quality, and is usually a subsidiary constituent in remedies.

Bael tree
Aegle marmelos (L.) Corrêa; *Rutaceae*

This small to medium-sized deciduous tree with long, sharp thorns is indigenous to the western Himalayas and dry forests of India, but is now cultivated in eastern India and on the islands of Indonesia. The fruits are round to oval in shape, between 5 and 12 centimetres in size, and their

Cumin
Cuminum cyminum L.; *Umbelliferae*

Cumin is an ancient herbal remedy that has been found in Egyptian tombs. It is indigenous to the Mediterranean, and mainly cultivated in Egypt, Morocco and Syria, as well as India, North America and Chile. The plant belongs to the same family as coriander and caraway. As with these, it is the fruits that are used but, unlike coriander, they ripen into two characteristic, slightly curved, greyish seed-fruits. Cumin was hardly known in former times, but it has established itself as a common ingredient in Western cooking through the increasing popularity of Indian and North African cuisine.

TIBETAN NAME AND CHARACTERIZATION

In Tibet cumin is known as *ziradkarpo* (tchira-karpo). The fruits are used. Tibetan classification ascribes to cumin the taste sphere sharp and sweet, and the active force hot. It is effective for *badkan* disorders and digestive problems. The same name is given to a yellow variety of cumin, which derives from a yellow flowering plant.

Indian sea-grape

Ephedra gerardiana Wall. Ex Stapf; Ephedrae

The Indian sea-grape is indigenous to northern India, Kashmir and Afghanistan, where it prefers dry locations. The plant grows into a small, almost vertical bush, whose appearance is reminiscent of horsetail. Dark green, cylindrical twigs sprout from stem-nodes 1 to 2 millimetres thick. The plant has a male and female form. The very small flowers develop into edible, oval fruit.

TIBETAN NAME AND CHARACTERIZATION

This plant is called *mtseldum* (tse-dum), and only the twigs are used for medicinal purposes. The medicinal substance obtained from it has a bitter taste and a cooling active force. It is effective at stopping bleeding and is used for various kinds of 'fever'.

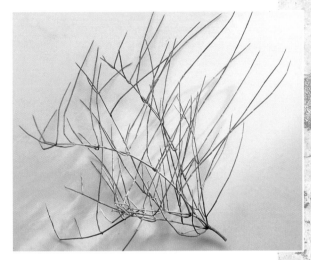

Only the twigs of the Indian sea-grape are used medicinally.

Tamala cinnamon

Cinnamomum tamala (Buch.-Ham.) Nees & Eberm.; Lauraceae

The Tamala cinnamon tree comes from the Himalayas, where it grows at altitudes of 900 to 2,400 metres. This evergreen tree, growing up to 7.5 metres high, has a coarse, dark brown to black bark, and foliage of oval, lancet-shaped, smooth leaves. In India the leaves are used.

TIBETAN NAME AND CHARACTERIZATION

The Tibetan name for this plant is *drizhimloma* (dri-shim-lo-ma). Tamala cinnamon is fragrant and has a hot and sharp active force.

Medical compounds

The three fruits

'*bras bu gsum* (dre-bu-sum)

'*Brasbugsum* is the compound name for the mixture of medicines made from the three myrobalan fruits – the *chebula, bellirica* and *emblica myrobalans*. It often features in remedies and is also a remedy in its own right (prepared by boiling), and known as '*brasbusgumthung* (dre-bu-sum-thang). It counteracts *rlung* disorders.

The three sharp medicines
Tshabagsum (tsa-wa-sum)

The three medicines black pepper, long pepper and ginger are also often combined in remedies, and given the single name *Tshabagsum*. This remedy has a sharp taste and a hot active force.

The three fragrant medicines
drigsum (dri-sum)

This fragrant mixture consists of cinnamon, Tamala cinnamon and cardamom. It has the active forces hot, sharp and oily, stimulates digestion and appetite and is said to be effective against chronic sneezing and parasite infestation.

On the art of herb gathering

The ancient medical texts list specific requirements for gathering plants, right down to the smallest details, such as the best time of year. Roots, bark and sap or resin are gathered in the early spring; fruit, blossoms, leaves and stems in the late spring; and seeds during the monsoon. Astrological criteria also play a role: particularly favourable days for gathering herbs lie between the 7th and 15th day of the lunar month, during the phase of the waxing moon. Weather conditions must also be observed. Furthermore, the plants must be thriving and undamaged, and be growing in a favourable location. Plants for treating hot illnesses should be gathered from north-facing slopes and plants that are good for cold illnesses from south-facing slopes and valleys. Instructions for

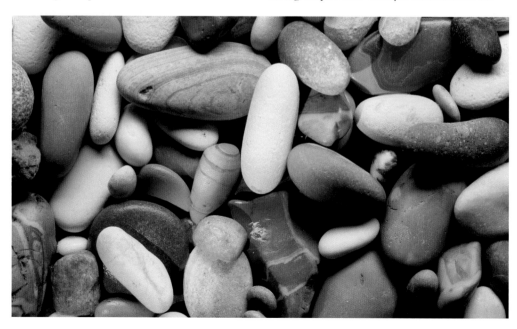

handling before drying and processing are also stipulated. In medical schools, the pupils gather medicinal herbs alongside their teachers. In summer these groups go on expeditions into the mountains lasting several weeks or even months, just as they did a hundred years ago, to pursue plants *in situ*.

Plant-gathering is accompanied by special rites: the mantras of the Medicine Buddha are regularly chanted as work begins. Accompanying prayers are meant to guarantee that medicinal plants are plucked in the right spiritual attitude of compassion.

However, the huge increase in international interest in Asiatic herbal medicine seems to be affecting the unspoiled plant kingdom of the Himalayas. Because of great demand there is now a shortage of raw materials, and in some regions too many plants are being harvested. Awareness that they are destroying their own herbal resources is now forcing Tibetan doctors and botanists to seek alternatives. In the Tibetan Medical and Astrological Institute at Dharamsala, trials are being undertaken to grow wild Himalayan plants in a greenhouse. No results are available as yet. Other attempts to cultivate medicinal plants in the Darjeeling mountains have apparently been unsuccessful. Considering how swiftly species of plant are vanishing from the face of the Earth each year, these small attempts seem mere drops in the ocean. Western initiatives are probably required as well – for, after all, it is the 'civilized world' that has helped to create this situation.

The Constitution Types

If you ask a Tibetan about his energy or constitution type, he will be able to tell you without a moment's hesitation. In the same way as we classify our zodiac signs, he defines himself according to energy type. The basis for this classification is the doctrine of the three bodily energies *rlung*, *mkhrispa* and *badkan*. Each person belongs from birth to one of these three fundamental energies, or to a combination of them:

1. *rlung*
2. *mkhrispa*
3. *badkan*
4. *rlung/mkhrispa*
5. *rlung/badkan*
6. *mkhrispa/badkan*
7. *rlung/mkhrispa/badkan*

Knowing a person's constitutional type is the fundamental prerequisite for every Tibetan treatment. It can be judged most precisely by means of pulse diagnosis but if you don't have a Tibetan doctor or healer on hand to undertake this, you can consult the checklist on pages 78 and 79.

Checking the test

To be sure that you have given the right answers, it is worth asking someone who knows you very well to check and perhaps correct it. Where there is any doubt, remember that the preferences, characteristics or qualities towards which you most commonly tend are the important thing. Of course there are always times or phases when we react untypically. With counter-checking this test has 70 per cent accuracy.

To ascertain the result, count how many times you have given an answer from the *rlung*, *mkhrispa* or *badkan* column. Then enter the results as follows:

rlung	....	per cent
mkhrispa	....	per cent
badkan	....	per cent

Depending on the percentages, you can now classify yourself as one of the seven constitution types. Here are some examples:

• 70 per cent *rlung*, 20 per cent *badkan*, 10 per cent *mkhrispa*: your constitution type is *rlung*
• 50 per cent *rlung*, 50 per cent *badkan*: you are a classic *rlung/badkan* combination
• 45 per cent *rlung*, 55 per cent *mkhrispa*: your energy type is *rlung/mkhrispa*, with a slight preponderance of *mkhrispa*
• 40 per cent *mkhrispa*, 60 per cent *badkan*: you are a *badkan/mkhrispa* type with a preponderance of *badkan*
• 33 per cent *mkhrispa*, 37 per cent *badkan*, 30 per cent *rlung*: you correspond to the *badkan/mkhrispa/rlung* type

How the constitution arises

A person's fundamental constitution remains the same all his life. It is established in the womb and is determined by the energy type of sperm and egg, as well as by the way the mother conducts herself and eats during pregnancy. For example, if sperm and egg are chiefly *mkhrispa*, or if the mother eats mainly sharp and hot foods, which emphasize *mkhrispa*, the child will be born with a *mkhrispa* constitution. However, the dominance of *mkhrispa* does not always remain equally strong. There are many nuances in the interplay of energies. At different stages of life, at different seasons and even within a single day, one or another energy will manifest more strongly – similar to the way our desires and needs alter with changing circumstances, although we remain basically the same.

The three energies or principles are the basis of a person's mind and body. They determine his character and instincts, his likes and dislikes, and his manner of reacting to and thinking about things. Knowing your type, and determining your diet, behaviour, lifestyle, surroundings and biorhythms accordingly, is the best means of avoiding illness. The typologies also indicate our physical, emotional and mental weak points and vulnerabilities. And once we know these we can take steps to counteract harmful influences.

The three basic types

Rlung: vulture, raven, fox

Physically these people tend to be small, delicate and refined, weak and unmuscular. They often stoop forwards, sometimes have rounded shoulders and prominent joints, which easily break. Their skin colour tends to go bluish, and they cope very badly with cold and wind. *Rlung* types also dislike the night-time, twilight and extreme heat. They like sour, bitter, sweet and hot things. They often yawn and tend to have a dry mouth, and vacillate between hunger and lack of appetite. They sleep lightly and are easily woken.

According to Tibetan lore, *rlung* people have the nature of vulture, raven and fox, and their energies are classified under the elements air and space. They are said to enjoy laughing, singing and talking, and tend to be chatterboxes. But they also like quarrelling, are cowardly and have a poor memory. Typically they are unpredictable, restless, 'windy' spirits. They are often anxious, easily worried, and many thoughts pass through their heads. The Tibetans say that *rlung* types do not grow very old or very rich, but of course this depends a great deal on their race, way of life and circumstances.

From a medical perspective, *rlung* people have an 'unstable digestive heat'. The digestive organs are their most vulnerable region. The large intestine is most at risk, and any stress quickly affects their stomach. The heart is also vulnerable in this type, and they suffer more frequently than others from vascular disorders and stress-related illnesses. Overall the *rlung* type has cold, unstable and very changeable properties, which can vacillate from cold to hot. They are cured and brought back into balance by everything that grounds them and makes them heavier, warmer and more stable. OPTIMUM DIET: warm, protein-rich food that is not easily digested – for instance, meat broth and heavy, cooked foods such as leguminous vegetables combined with grains; couscous with chick-peas or rice with beans. *Rlung* copes well with sweet, sour and salty foods, as well as dairy products and mild spices such as cloves or turmeric. They take well to sweet desserts such as puddings or pastries, and a glass of wine with a meal will do no harm either.

TO BE AVOIDED: extremely bitter, sharp foods, raw fruit and vegetables, especially salads made from acidic vegetables such as tomatoes; cold dishes such as half-frozen puddings or ice-cream, and ice-cold drinks; foods that are too spicy (chilli); stimulants such as coffee; and any kind of drug.

OPTIMUM LIFESTYLE: a beautiful and peaceful environment, no emotional stress, no tension in the surroundings, warmth of every kind; well-heated rooms, warm clothing, pleasant music, yellow colours, harmonious conversation with friends. *Rlung* people should immediately respond to their body's every need: for instance, going to the toilet immediately they feel the need, not suppressing their yawns and eating the moment they feel hungry.

Mkhrispa: tiger and monkey

Physically these people tend to be medium-sized and muscular, with fair hair and light skin. They are often hungry and thirsty, have a good metabolism, good digestion and a healthy appetite; and their body reacts swiftly to even mild laxatives. It is noticeable that this type sweats easily and has a strong body odour.

Which type are you?

Tick one box from each of three possible answers.

CHARACTERISTIC	rlung	mkhrispa	badkan
BODY SIZE	very tall or very short	average	small
BUILD	delicate	average	heavy-limbed
TENDENCY TO	low weight	ideal weight	overweight
SHOULDERS	narrow	average	broad
HIPS	narrow	average	broad
CHEST	flat	normally developed	fully developed
SKIN	rough and dry	shiny	soft and smooth
SKIN	cold	warm	cool
SKIN	brownish	reddish	white
SWEAT	little, odourless	much, strong odour	normal, pleasant
HAIR	dry	tends to be greasy	oily
HAIR	curly	straight	wavy
HAIR	average	fine	strong
HAIR	dandruffy	soon goes grey	healthy
HAIR COLOUR	black	blond/red/light brown	brown to dark brown
FACIAL SKIN	wrinkled	reddish	smooth
NAILS	break easily	flexible	strong
NAILS	bluish	pinkish	pale
EYES	small	average	large
EYES	dry	red	moist
EYES	restless	penetrating	shining
EYES	blue, grey	bright	pale
NOSE	small	average	large
NOSE	narrow, straight	straight, pointed	fleshy, blunt
TEETH	small, crooked	medium, straight	large, straight
LIPS	narrow, dry	average, red	full, moist
FINGERS	slender, long	pointed, medium-sized	broad, short
FEET	small, narrow	medium	large, wide
FEET AND HANDS	cold and dry	hot, sweaty	cool, damp
VEINS	easily visible	faintly visible	invisible
FAT LAYER	around the waist	evenly distributed	around thighs and bottom
MUSCULATURE	poorly developed	athletic	well-developed, fat
ACTIVITY	hyperactive	normally active	little active
GAIT	tending to quick	medium	tending to slow
ENERGY	quick energy, little persistence	energy and persistence	slow energy, but persistent

CHARACTERISTIC	*rlung*	*mkhrispa*	*badkan*
VOICE	weak, quiet, rough	high, piercing	pleasant, deep
SLEEP	light and easily disturbed	deep, profound	long, sound
DREAMS	anxious, about flying and leaping	passionate, of colours and fire	romantic, about water and sea
SPEECH	quick, chatterbox	clear, eloquent	peaceful, melodious
MENSTRUATION	irregular, painful	regular, strong	regular, normal
URINE	little	much, burning	moderate, cloudy
STOOL	dry, dark, hard	oily, yellowish, loose	solid, well-formed
DIGESTION	sensitive, easily upset	good	bad
CREATIVITY	creative, imaginative	inventive, technical/scientific	mostly in a professional context
CONCENTRATION	poor	excellent	moderately good
MEMORY	good short-term, bad long-term	excellent	long-term good, short-term bad
DECISION-MAKING	problematic	quick, sure	slow, careful
COMPREHENSION	superficial	quick	slow, thorough
BELIEF	inconstant, changing like the wind	fanatic, intense	unwavering
WAY WITH MONEY	wastes money	methodical	saves for food
MAINLY SPENDS ON	trivial things	luxuries, enjoyment	investments
BUSINESS SENSE	bad, but has good ideas	good salesman, good at implementing ideas	excellent as a manager
I AM MORE	anxious, fearful	courageous, impulsive	loving
I AM MORE	shy	jealous	considerate
I AM MORE	gullible	ambitious	lethargic
I AM MORE	chaotic	irritable	peace-loving
I AM MORE	nervous	envious	yielding
I AM MORE	depressive	provocative	sentimental
I AM MORE	neurotic	charismatic	conservative
I AM MORE	no confidence	egotistic	self-content
I AM MORE	intuitive	practical	dreamy
I AM MORE	unstable	quick to anger	generous
I AM MORE	over-sensitive	intolerant	miserly
TENDENCY TO	nervousness	stomach problems	much mucus
TENDENCY TO	bad circulation	high blood pressure	high cholesterol
TENDENCY TO	rheumatism/arthritis	acne	colds
TENDENCY TO	stiff limbs	gum/nose bleeding	breathing problems
THIRST	changeable	a great deal	little
APPETITE	changeable	very good	little
I HATE	all forms of cold	strong heat	can cope with either

The *mkhrispa* type's weak points are liver, gall bladder and small intestine. For this reason, they often tend to suffer from complaints of the upper abdomen. They are also prone to 'hot' infectious diseases, inflammations and febrile infections. These most often occur during dry spells and hot weather, as well as at midday, midnight and in the autumn.

Mkhrispa is assigned to the element of fire, and this explains this type's typical characteristics. They are extremely quick on the uptake, clear in their thinking and very convincing and compelling. They are bold, courageous, self-aware, adventurous, acrobatic, impetuous and daring – similar to tigers and monkeys. The other side of their fiery temperament is their quick anger and jealousy, and temper tantrums. To the fire-related *mkhrispa* type is ascribed the properties of hot, dry and oily. It needs to be balanced by moisture and cold – in diet, climate and medical treatment.

OPTIMUM DIET: raw food and fruit of all kinds and varieties, cool drinks, cold water, ending a meal with half-frozen desserts of ice-cream or fruit.

TO BE AVOIDED: alcohol and coffee, too much meat, too much oil and fat, strong spices.

OPTIMUM LIFESTYLE: damp, cool climate, winter temperatures. The perfect location would be a waterfall surrounded by shady trees. Mental and physical peace counteracts much of the *mkhrispa* type's fire. They shouldn't go on holiday to hot places, but to cool, northern regions. Hot baths and saunas should be avoided, as well as stress, sudden energetic physical work, intense mental activity and in general too many activities at once. Sunbathing is thought to be particularly bad for them. If possible this 'hot' energy type should take a lot of cold showers and cold water therapies.

Badkan: lion and bull

The *badkan* type is very strongly built, has a well-developed 'cool' body with thick skin. Their joints are often almost invisible. These types usually have a very erect posture, are robust and hardy. They have a good constitution and are regarded as resilient. They can endure hunger and thirst for several days on end. A striking feature of such types is their 'blessed'

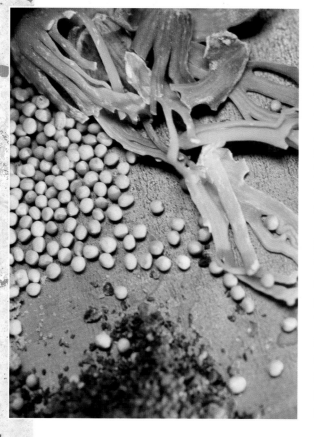

sleep: they sleep deeply and soundly and when things are not going well for them they develop a strong need to sleep. Their 'digestion warmth' tends to be weak and slow, and their digestion sluggish in consequence. They like eating sharp and bitter foods. *Badkan* belongs to the element of earth (*ba*) and water (*kan*). These determine the type's weak points: water-retention (oedema), swellings in the face, hands and feet; and also susceptibility to the typical 'mucus' illnesses such as asthma or blocked sinuses. Lungs, respiratory tract, kidneys, stomach and spleen are all vulnerable. A further problem is their tendency to corpulence, which can lead to metabolic diseases such as diabetes.

By nature, *badkan* people are tolerant, peaceful, friendly and altruistic; also loyal, considerate and obedient. They tend to be shy. The Tibetans assign the animals lion and bull to these characteristics. It is also said of *badkan* types that they grow very old and very rich, but as with the *rlung* type this should be taken with a pinch of salt. *Badkan* has the properties of cool and moist, so diet and therapy should have the properties of warm and dry.

OPTIMUM DIET: cooked, warm food without sauce, such as lightly cooked vegetables with fresh herbs. A good medicine is ginger powder – either as tea or condiment.

TO BE AVOIDED: everything moist and cold. Cold salad, raw food, fatty foods, sauces, fried foods, soups and starchy vegetables such as leguminous foods. Root vegetables, even when cooked, have a cold effect within the body. It is better to drink a glass of boiled water after eating rather than drinking too much with the meal.

OPTIMUM LIFESTYLE: dry, warm climate. A lot of daily activity. Exercise before meals and don't nap in the middle of the day. As a physical exercise for the *badkan* type, Tibetan doctors recommend prostrations, as practised by Buddhists when they are walking round holy sites.

The four combination types

People in whom two energies dominate, or in whom all three energies are evenly distributed, should regulate their behaviour and lifestyle accordingly. Here are some points of reference:

rlung/badkan – cool and changeable

This type is often of medium size, slim, well-built and prone to nervousness, but by nature usually tolerant and somewhat lethargic. Certain characteristics indicate a dominance of one or the other energy; and recommendations are made accordingly. Big weight swings suggest a *rlung* dominance, while constant weight is a *badkan* characteristic. A fundamental principle here is that all cold intensifies *badkan* energy, and this in turn increases the changeable *rlung* energy, which intensifies all other energies. Thus warm food, medicines and locations are recommended. As far as diet and lifestyle are concerned, this type can choose at will from recommendations for *rlung* and *badkan*. But where there are health problems, they should take the medicines for *badkan* complaints yet adjust diet and lifestyle for the *rlung* type. In specific terms this could mean not eating too heavily, not drinking coffee or light foods, and drinking a lot of boiled, warm water. Sesame oil, honey and fish are recommended. Strongly built *rlung/badkan* people, who are prone to nervousness, should fast often to counter this, and take care to move and exercise a lot. Fasting is far less tolerable to slim and peaceful types.

rlung/mkhrispa – the 'hot' personality

Many people of this combination type are physically very strong and active, and full of energy. They tend to be self-aware, but the heat quality makes them prone to temper and aggression. The *rlung* aspects of their nature also make them restless and changeable in their opinions. They often make promises which they do not keep. They like talking about themselves, and are prone to headaches and dizziness. People of this type usually have a good digestive heat. If *mkhrispa* dominates, they sweat a good deal; when *rlung* dominates they are sometimes constipated. In this combination, *rlung* intensifies the prevalent tendency – in this case heat. This means that, in principle, cool foods, medicines and locations are recommended: no sun, no hot spices. When there are health problems, *rlung* also intensifies the hot energy, and thus inflammations, fever and febrile infections easily arise. Fever is regarded as a classic *rlung/mkhrispa* illness. *Rlung* symbolizes the cold (shivering) that is experienced before the outbreak of fever, and the weakness and

weariness afterwards. At the outset, when they are shivering and feeling miserable, the patient should eat *rlung* foods and take medicine suited to *mkhrispa*. If the temperature still continues to rise, only *mkhrispa* foods and medicines should be taken.

mkhrispa/badkan – a hot-cold combination

In the West we would normally think of such a person as contradictory and difficult, because of the combination of these two opposite characteristics of hot and cold. But Tibetan medicine sees things quite differently. If both poles are equally strong, harmony results. The *mkhrispa/badkan* type is regarded as generally harmonious. For instance, he can have a thoughtful manner and a steady, trustworthy (*badkan*) nature; and nevertheless be very physically active (*mkhrispa*). Another combination is a fiery and aggressive (*mkhrispa*) temperament hiding within a rather lethargic and corpulent (*badkan*) body.

Everything should be in moderation for this combination type – diet, medicines and location should be neither too hot nor too cold. In real terms this might mean having warm but not hot baths, drinking lukewarm drinks, living in a moderate climate, taking care not to go out in the baking sun and avoiding over-spiced foods. The choice of diet should take an individual's digestion into consideration. If the digestion functions well, cooling *mkhrispa* foods are preferable; sluggish digestion, on the other hand, requires warming *badkan* fare.

mkhrispa/rlung/badkan – the epitome of harmony

This combination type composed of all three energies is very rare. It is regarded as the most balanced, however, because it unites all three principles in a harmonious whole. According to Tibetan medicine, this combination gives rise to an ideal personality: a balanced person who does not fall seriously ill either in mind or body, and who has sufficient capacities at his disposal to achieve his aims. The great quality of this triple energy combination seems to lie in its flexibility and ability to adapt. People of this type are extremely resilient and deal very well with stress. They can master difficult situations. As far as preferred diet, medicines and lifestyle are concerned, the *mkhrispa/rlung/badkan* type can adapt himself to external circumstances such as the weather or season, and follow his needs accordingly. Further points to consider are the person's digestive heat: if this is strong, *mkhrispa* diet and lifestyle are recommended; if changeable, *rlung* recommendations are helpful; and in the case of sluggish digestion, the *badkan* suggestions should be followed.

Severe and slight illnesses

Corresponding to their weak points, the *rlung* energy type tends to *rlung* illnesses, the *mkhrispa* type to *mkhrispa* illnesses; and the *badkan* type to *badkan* illnesses. Such complaints are usually severe and prolonged because they issue from the core of a person's nature. But there are also forms of illness which do not accord with the constitutional type. For instance, a *rlung/badkan* type can develop *mkhrispa* symptoms of illness, the *mkhrispa* type can develop *rlung* complaints, and the *rlung* type can develop *mkhrispa/badkan* illnesses. Such disorders tend to be less severe, because their symptoms are more 'external' and do not arise from a person's innate nature. To treat such illnesses, doctors prescribe medicines determined by the energy type, and a diet suited to the hot or cold nature of the symptoms. For instance, if the cool *rlung/badkan* type develops hot *mkhrispa* symptoms such as fever, the doctor will diagnose this as a cold illness with hot symptoms, prescribing pills for *rlung* or *badkan*, but a *mkhrispa* diet. This is just one example of the great differentiation that is possible in Tibetan medicine.

SELF-TREATMENT A-Z

Arthritis

DISTURBED BODY ENERGY: *badkan*, often also *rlung*.
DISTURBED ELEMENTS: water and earth, possibly also air.
Many Tibetans suffer from arthritis due to the extreme cold in the Himalayas.

DIETARY RECOMMENDATIONS

AVOID: old, rancid, sour, oily and heavy foods, which are 'poison' to arthritis. Salt, potatoes and cabbage are also bad.
RECOMMENDED: rice, roasted barley, peas, dandelion leaves, buttermilk and yoghurt made from cow's milk; cold, boiled water;

light foods, and wine with a little honey. Condiments and seasonings that can be used generously: cinnamon, ginger, honey, pomegranate seeds, long pepper, saffron, coriander and black pepper.

For chronic arthritis, the following radish cure is an extremely successful Tibetan remedy:

In the evening, peel a Tibetan radish root (you can also use white radish), cut it into small pieces and wrap it in a clean cotton cloth. Then wring the cloth until it exudes radish juice. Collect the juice in a glass and spoon off the bubbles that have collected on the top. Wring the cloth out several times, each time collecting the juice in the glass and spooning off the bubbles. Then leave the juice to stand overnight in a cool, dark place. The next morning you can add a little ground fenugreek to taste, and then drink it on an empty stomach.

LIFESTYLE
AVOID: everything that makes the body cold; in winter, never go outside with inadequate clothing. Don't lie down in fierce sun in summer; don't sit close to a source of heat, or go to sleep during the daytime. Take care to avoid wet or damp places or environments.
RECOMMENDED: gymnastics; keeping the feet, hips and thighs warm at all times.

THERAPIES
Physiotherapy.
Bathing in hot springs (also thermal baths). Tibetans add certain medicinal herbs to the bathwater: *shugpa, balu, tsadh, khenpa, yombu*. These plants only grow in the Himalayas and are known by their Tibetan names.

Asthma

DISTURBED BODY ENERGY: *badkan*.
DISTURBED ELEMENTS: water and earth.
Bronchial asthma is chiefly attributable to *badkan* disturbances, while allergic asthma arises from *rlung* problems. In cases of allergic asthma, you should avoid anything that reinforces *rlung* energy.

DIETARY RECOMMENDATIONS
AVOID: cold foods, cold drinks, bananas, avocado, fried and roasted foods, ice-cream.
REDUCE CONSUMPTION OF: dairy products, sweet and oily foods, white bread, products made with white flour.
RECOMMENDED: warm food, boiled water (especially after meals), ginger tea, goat's milk, wholegrain products.

LIFESTYLE
RECOMMENDED: breathing exercises, jogging, swimming, fasting (if overweight), eating little and often.
AVOID: eating too much, working in the sun, stress, stale or polluted air.

THERAPIES
The following gentle heat-cure, mentioned in the *rGyudbzhi*, is very helpful:
1 teaspoon sesame oil
½ teaspoon ground nutmeg
½ teaspoon yellow cumin
1 piece thin cotton dressing
1 piece of thread
Mix the nutmeg and cumin, wrap the mixture in the dressing then form a small ball and tie it with thread. Heat up the sesame oil and dip the ball into it until it is saturated with hot oil. Then place the ball on the acupressure point in the middle of the chest exactly midway between the

nipples, and leave it there until it has cooled. If necessary dip it in hot oil again and repeat.

Cupping therapy on the back and chest is also recommended but should only be carried out by a doctor or therapist.

Bronchitis

DISTURBED BODY ENERGY: *mkhrispa, badkan.*

DISTURBED ELEMENTS: fire, water, earth.
Tibetan medicine defines bronchitis as a combined *mkhrispa/badkan* illness, because of the simultaneous inflammation and mucus production.

DIETARY RECOMMENDATIONS

AVOID: fried foods, fats, 'warmth-inducing' meat such as chicken, lamb or pork, mature cheese and cured meats such as salami.

RECOMMENDED: eat a lot of fruit, especially grapes. Use spices and herbs such as saffron, liquorice root, sandalwood, cloves, cinnamon, safflower and the Tibetan myrobalan *Arura terminalia*. Ensure that the food you eat is fresh, especially butter and milk. (This piece of advice may seem strange to us, but the Tibetans often cook meat that is no longer completely fresh, or use older, sometimes rancid butter.)

There is a Tibetan tea to alleviate bronchitis, consisting of a plant called *tarbu* together with buckthorn (or sandthorn) fruits. Both these ingredients are contained in herb pills for bronchitis called 'Tsowo 8', 'Tsowo 25', 'Pangyen 15', 'Chugang 25' and 'Lingun 11'. Warning: it is not advisable to take these pills without consulting a Tibetan doctor, because they need to be individually prescribed according to the patient's energy type.

To make a tea from herbs available in the UK: mix equal parts of ground cloves, liquorice root and cinnamon. Brew a teaspoonful of this mixture in a cup of water.

LIFESTYLE

RECOMMENDED: for chronic bronchitis, you should adopt a regime of regular fasting, breathing exercises (especially in the morning), and occasional intestinal cleansing with laxatives (consult your doctor about this).

THERAPIES

Tibetan doctors treat acute bronchitis by cupping.

Colds

DISTURBED BODY ENERGY: *rlung/mkhrispa.*
DISTURBED ELEMENTS: air, fire.
In Tibetan medicine, a cold is regarded as a disturbance of energy and the immune system. The most important cure is to avoid everything cold, otherwise *rlung* energy increases still further.

DIETARY RECOMMENDATIONS

AVOID: cold foods, radish, garlic.
REDUCE CONSUMPTION OF: onions.
RECOMMENDED: boiled, warm water, warm foods.

A daily cup of 'Sorig-Tea', made from Tibetan herbs, also helps combat colds. It is produced in the Medical and Astrological Institute in Dharamsala, and can be supplied by mail order (*see page 157*).

LIFESTYLE

AVOID: cold showers, clothing that is not warm enough.

RECOMMENDED: Champa-dance. This is a dance similar to the lama dances, in which the whole body is thoroughly shaken, and the body's defence mechanisms are shaken awake.

Constipation

DISTURBED BODY ENERGIES: usually *rlung* and *badkan*.
DISTURBED ELEMENTS: air, earth. Water, particularly in the digestive system.

DIETARY RECOMMENDATIONS

AVOID: cold and starchy foods, such as bananas, sugar, white flour. Fatty meat, heavy foods and eating too much.
REDUCE CONSUMPTION OF: white rice.
RECOMMENDED: foods made from whole grains, wholegrain rice, yoghurt, sweetened tea with milk drunk before breakfast in the mornings (Indians drink this every morning to stimulate digestion), papaya, linseed (*sarma*), boiled, warm water.

LIFESTYLE

Fasting is a proven means of cleansing and stimulating the intestine.

THERAPIES

Enemas are the best therapy for constipation. Only warm water should be used.
Moxa therapy has been effectively used for stomach pains in the navel region.
'Shiru' is a tried and tested Tibetan herb pill for sluggish digestion but it should only be taken after consultation with a Tibetan doctor. The daily dose is three pills half an hour before breakfast and three pills half an hour after supper. The pills are ground into coarse pieces in a mortar, and swallowed with warm, boiled water.

Diarrhoea

DISTURBED BODY ENERGY: *rlung/mkhrispa*.
DISTURBED ELEMENT: air.
This is usually a cold illness.

DIETARY RECOMMENDATIONS

AVOID: all foods with a cooling effect.
RECOMMENDED: a small glass of herbal schnapps/spirits. If the complaint is due to weak digestion, either fasting or the following porridge drink will help:

Roast a few oatflakes and boil in a cup of water. Add a few chunks of tender lamb and a pinch of ginger powder; and then drink it like a soup. Then drink a good quantity of warm, boiled water.

Another useful recipe is 'rice-porridge':

Cook 1 teaspoon of rice in two cups of water until soft. Mash the rice to a porridge consistency, add some sheep's milk butter and season with a little salt and sugar to taste.

LIFESTYLE

AVOID: everything that makes the body cold or cools it down, such as sitting in draughts or walking around naked or with too little clothing.
RECOMMENDED: place a strip of animal fleece or a warm cloth around the stomach.

THERAPIES

If the complaint is due to a cold illness of the intestine, gentle heat therapy will help. The Tibetans heat a flat stone in a stove and place it on the navel.
In the case of heavy diarrhoea, there is a danger that the body will become dehydrated. To combat this, the *rGyudbzhi* describes a treatment called White therapy, involving an ancient Tibetan formula

('white' refers to the milk): *Melt 1 teaspoon of butter made from sheep's milk, add 4 teaspoons roasted barley-meal (tsampa), and then boil well with ½ cup milk. Add 1 large pinch ground ginger and 1 large pinch rock salt, making a paste out of the mixture. Eat this paste in the mornings and evenings, but prepare it freshly each time. You can add ½ teaspoon sugar to improve the taste!*

There is a Tibetan herb pill that counteracts diarrhoea, called 'Sedu 5'. Ask a Tibetan doctor about this.

Eczema

DISTURBED BODY ENERGIES: *rlung/badkan.*
DISTURBED ELEMENTS: water, earth.
Most eczema-type skin problems have internal causes and are chronic. These are classic *badkan* themes. Skin disorders tend to be *rlung* problems. Both together give the *rlung/badkan* combination.

DIETARY RECOMMENDATIONS

AVOID: sour or acidic foods and drinks such as vinegar, chutney, eggs, fermented fruit or vegetables, bottled fruit, alcohol, beer, mature cheese, hot spices, pork.
REDUCE CONSUMPTION OF: fats, meat.
RECOMMENDED: fresh fruit.

LIFESTYLE

AVOID: stress.
RECOMMENDED: keep the affected areas of the skin dry, don't bathe for too long and don't work up too much sweat, for instance during sport or in the sauna.

THERAPIES

'Sorig-ointment' cream was specially developed at the Tibetan Medical and Astrological Institute at Dharamsala to

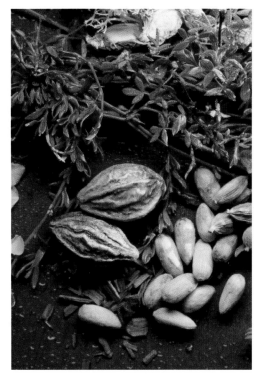

combat eczema and skin rashes. This ointment contains 12 Tibetan medicinal herbs and is said to be extremely effective. It is safe to use on weeping or suppurating skin regions. Apply to affected areas mornings and evenings.

As well as this ointment, Tibetan doctors usually prescribe three kinds of pill to treat eczema. They are called 'Gurgum 13', 'Pokar 10', and 'Nilar'. Take 3 'Gurgum 13' in the morning, 3 'Pokar 10' at midday and 3 'Nilar' in the evening.

Fatigue

DISTURBED BODY ENERGIES: *rlung, badkan.*
DISTURBED ELEMENTS: air, water, earth.
Chronic tiredness is a Western illness. Tibetans are not familiar with the lack of motivation resulting from stress and

pressure to achieve, and they are rarely subject to work-related stress. Tibetan doctors diagnose these symptoms as too little *rlung* and too much *badkan*. Body heat is reduced, so the sufferer has cold hands and feet; there are often digestive problems because of the linked reduction in digestive heat. Symptoms of excess *badkan* include a feeling of heaviness and weakness, and difficulties in breathing and concentrating.

DIETARY RECOMMENDATIONS

AVOID: garlic and onions, milk products in the morning, eating too much at once.

REDUCE CONSUMPTION OF: fats, salt, sweet things, cold drinks, cold food.

RECOMMENDED: eat five small meals through the course of the day, making sure that you do not over-indulge so that you still feel fresh after a meal. Drink a lot of warm, boiled water, eat warming spices such as ginger. Stick to a vegetarian diet with plenty of fresh fruit (but not bananas) and cooked green vegetables. Fish is allowed.

LIFESTYLE

AVOID: working at night, taking work home with you from the office, working overtime. Massages are not necessarily a good idea because they further reduce the already diminished *rlung* energy. Even if you find it difficult, avoid sleeping during the day, for this strengthens the already over-dominant *badkan* energy, and you will feel even more tired than you did before.

RECOMMENDED: the most important remedies are peace and relaxation. Keep the weekend as a time to relax, plan a recovery programme and cure, notice and give in to your physical needs; take care to have warm feet, and to be always warm in winter.

Plan times for general relaxation and gentle meditative practice (*see pages 116 to 120*). All these exercises require you not to talk too much but to remain as 'centred' in yourself as you can. Gentle (unpressurized) movement such as jogging is also good.

THERAPIES

For fatigue, Tibetan doctors prescribe the herbal medicines 'Sedu 5' or 'Kundey'.

Gall-stones

DISTURBED ENERGY: *mkhrispa*.

DISTURBED ELEMENT: fire.

Gall-stones are very painful. Sufferers have pains to the right of the navel and, in the case of large stones, in the chest and back as well. Sometimes the skin and eyes take on a yellowish tinge.

DIETARY RECOMMENDATIONS

AVOID: it is very important not to eat too much at once; eat small, regular portions instead. If possible, give up salt, fat, oily foods, meat (especially chicken and pork) and eggs.

RECOMMENDED: oranges, lemons, apples, sugar-beet syrup. The following spices and herbs are beneficial: saffron, turmeric, safflower, barberry root and a Tibetan variety of tarantula called *Swertia chiryata*.

THERAPY

Tibetan doctors have found that smaller gall-stones disappear after patients take the herbal remedies 'Serdog 5', 'Serdog 11' and 'Triche 7'. A doctor's prescription is required for these pills.

Haemorrhoids

DISTURBED BODY ENERGY: usually *rlung*, sometimes *mkhrispa*.

DISTURBED ELEMENTS: wind, fire.

DIETARY RECOMMENDATIONS

AVOID: sharp spices such as chilli, foods of very sour taste, bananas.

REDUCE CONSUMPTION OF: oil, spices.

RECOMMENDED: drinking a lot of buttermilk, rice and cooked vegetables, and lentil and meat soup.

LIFESTYLE

AVOID: sitting down for long periods, riding, soft chairs, straining to pass stools, enemas for intestinal cleansing, constipation.

THERAPY

A much-praised Tibetan remedy for haemorrhoids is to drink as much buttermilk as possible. It is said that simple, non-bleeding haemorrhoids shrink as a result.

A frequently prescribed remedy for haemorrhoids is called 'Emblica ribes 9'.

SESAME THERAPY

Boil ½ cup rice in a pot with 2 cups water, until the water becomes white. Strain off the rice and use only the rice water. Add 1 teaspoon sugar, 5 teaspoons sesame seeds and 1 glass milk. Let the mixture boil for a while. Drink a full bowl of this warm mixture each day.

Headaches

DISTURBED BODY ENERGIES: *rlung* or *mkhrispa*.

DISTURBED ELEMENTS: air or fire.

Headaches due to *mkhrispa* originate in digestive problems, while *rlung*-type headaches are the consequence of general bodily weakness. *Rlung* headaches are often accompanied by dizziness and tinnitus, and sometimes people feel sick. In cases of low blood pressure they may even pass out. Sometimes the pain spreads as far down as the cheeks, and even the gums, and the nose can be blocked. Typical of this type of headache is that the whole head hurts, and there is no specific pain site.

Mkhrispa headaches derive from disturbances of the liver, digestion and gall bladder. Typical signs of this are feeling sick and a definite distaste for oily or fatty foods. Such people often develop yellowish skin and yellow eye-balls, and their whole head and body becomes hot. They are usually better at night than during the day. The whole head also hurts.

FOR RLUNG-TYPE HEADACHES

DIETARY RECOMMENDATIONS

RECOMMENDED: chicken broth, enriched with melted butter and spiced with coriander.

THERAPIES

NASAL THERAPY: add 1 to 2 drops of the essential oils of cinnamon and nutmeg in a cup of warm, boiled water; stir and use as nose-drops in both nostrils.

Acupressure at the temple-point of the head and at the two hollows of the temples (*see page 123*). Acupressure massage should, if possible, be performed with specially prepared massage butter. See the directions for massage and the recipe for massage butter on pages 126 and 127. Following this massage, Tibetan doctors recommend drinking some melted butter in hot milk, or a half cup of pure, melted butter. In severe cases, cauterization therapy might be performed (*see page 52*).

FOR MKHRISPA-TYPE HEADACHES

DIETARY RECOMMENDATIONS

AVOID: oily foods, animal fats.

RECOMMENDED: bitter foods of all kinds, such as bitter lettuces and vegetables (e.g. artichokes), herbs of bitter taste, yoghurt, buttermilk, cold water.

THERAPIES

Cold compresses on the forehead.
Pouring cold water over the head.
Lighting sandalwood incense sticks.
Mix 3 drops sandalwood essential oil with one dessertspoon of sesame oil, and rub this into the acupressure points mentioned under *rlung* headaches. Freshly melted butter is just as good.

NASAL THERAPY: *½ cup water, ½ teaspoon sugar, 1 large pinch saffron and 1 teaspoon fresh butter. Boil the water with the sugar for a short time, melt the butter in it and finally add the saffron (do not boil). Cool and use lukewarm as nosedrops.*

High blood pressure

DISTURBED BODY ENERGY: *rlung.*
DISTURBED ELEMENTS: air with fire symptoms.

DIETARY RECOMMENDATIONS

AVOID: salt, oily foods, fried foods, alcohol, coffee, tea.

REDUCE CONSUMPTION OF: meat (apart from beef and fish), butter, fats, ginger, liquorice, hot pepper, sharp spices.

RECOMMENDED: vegetarian food, fasting, cooling foods, garlic (reduces *rlung*), using a lot of nutmeg with food, tea from

(Tibetan) Arura fruits (*see* Plant Descriptions, *page 66*).

The following tea is very beneficial for high blood pressure:

Debu sumthang – a decoction of three fruits (rarely obtainable in Europe): Arura (*Terminalia chebula*), Kyuru (*Emblica officinalis*), Baru (*Terminalia belerica*). Mix equal portions of all three herbs. Put one teaspoon in a cup and add boiling water. Drink one cup each day. This tea has cooling properties, and may also be beneficial if it is taken for a high temperature or at the onset of a fever.

LIFESTYLE

AVOID: stress, long periods in the sun, saunas, washing your hair with hot water.

RECOMMENDED: cold showers, washing your hair in cool water, always keeping the head cool.

THERAPIES

Cupping with blood-letting, golden needle therapy, golden hammer, meditation, Tibetan yoga (*Kum Nye*).

For incense therapy, two types of incense sticks are suitable:

• *Lung-poe*, which should only be used in the evening because it is very relaxing and encourages sleep.

• The incense sticks used in monasteries, which contain heart-strengthening plant substances. Use one each morning and again in the evening.

Insomnia

DISTURBED BODY ENERGY: usually *rlung.*
DISTURBED ELEMENT: air.

DIETARY RECOMMENDATIONS

AVOID: coffee, cold foods such as lettuce or

raw food, hot pepper, chilli, too many sweet things.

RECOMMENDED: spices and herbs such as nutmeg, asafoetida, sesame, cinnamon, cumin, cloves, garlic and onions. A glass of red wine with the midday and evening meals, warm milk before going to bed, meat broth with chicken and lamb.

LIFESTYLE

Don't take work home with you from the office. Listen to harmonious, calming music, don't talk too much in the evening, avoid exasperating conversations, eat early in the evening. You can also recite mantras or meditate in the evening.

THERAPIES

Nutmeg butter massage in the evening (*see page 127 for recipe*).

GARLIC THERAPY: *make a broth from shoulder of lamb, lamb tail-bone and some rock salt. Put a bowl of this in a pot and boil two whole bulbs of garlic with it for at least ten minutes until they are soft. Mash and mix to form a paste. Add 1 teaspoon of fresh butter. Drink in the evening.*

WINE THERAPY: *1 glass of mature red wine, 1 teaspoon old butter made from sheep's milk, 1 teaspoon sugar beet molasses, 1 large pinch ground ginger. Boil all the ingredients well and drink warm.*

INCENSE THERAPY: *one hour before going to sleep, light a Tibetan anti-stress incense stick (*rlung-poe*).*

Liver strain

DISTURBED BODY ENERGY: *mkhrispa*
DISTURBED ELEMENT: fire
Analgesics, antibiotics and environmental pollutants place a strain on our system's central detoxifying organ. Typical symptoms of an overstrained liver include reddish (sometimes yellowish) eyes, pale, bluish face-colour, pains in the rib region and around the liver. Pains after eating, dry stools, swollen joints in the feet, yellowish temples, palms and soles of the feet, and sudden outbreaks of rage that can turn into depressive moods.

Please note: the following self-help measures are not sufficient on their own. It is essential to consult a doctor.

DIETARY RECOMMENDATIONS

AVOID: alcohol and fats, pork, chicken and lamb.

REDUCE CONSUMPTION OF: salt, all spices and seasonings (except saffron and cumin).

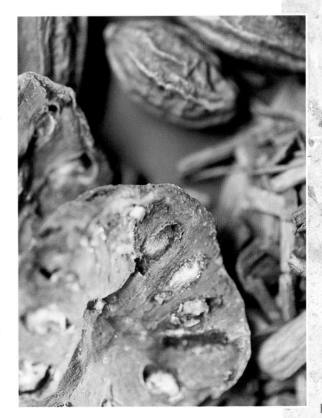

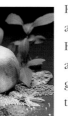

RECOMMENDED: saffron and cumin are said to sustain liver function. Herbs used in Tibetan medicine against liver disorders include gentian and barberry (particularly the root and inner bark).

Bitter-tasting vegetables are helpful, including chicory and other bitter lettuces. A good drink for the liver is sugar beet juice. Three glasses every day are thought to help at the beginning of a liver infection, if the skin turns yellow. Recommended fruits are: grapes, lemons, oranges, apples. Olives are also good for the liver.

THERAPIES

The precious pill 'Turquoise 25' cures liver problems. Ask a Tibetan doctor for a prescription. The pill can either be taken once a month at full or new moon, as a preventive measure against liver complaints; or, if liver disease already exists, once a week. There are certain stipulations when taking this pill; your doctor will advise.

Bloodletting carried out by a doctor is beneficial for liver strain.

Low blood pressure

DISTURBED BODY ENERGIES: *rlung* or *rlung/badkan*.
DISTURBED ELEMENTS: air, water, earth
Most people of the *rlung* or *rlung/badkan* energy types suffer from low blood pressure. Classic symptoms are feeling weak, getting tired easily and having a quiet voice. Such people often have dry skin. Tibetan doctors relate this disorder to the metabolism and absorption problems in the liver.

DIETARY RECOMMENDATIONS

AVOID: everything which increases *rlung* energy, such as pork, coffee, tea. Caffeine and tannin drinks disturb the energy system, by first raising blood pressure and then letting it fall lower again.
REDUCE CONSUMPTION OF: 'cold foods' (in the Tibetan sense of making the body cold), such as lettuce and fruit.
RECOMMENDED: foods of sour taste, radish, carrots, rice, green vegetables, eggs, lamb, fish, chicken. Warming drinks are good, such as ginger tea and all herbal liver remedies such as saffron, turmeric or safflower. If the patient does not suffer from oedema, he can take more salt than other people.
A TEA RECIPE: *grind pomegranate seeds, lemon peel and cardamom fruits in a mortar and mix equal parts. Use one teaspoon of the mixture per cup. A good drink for the morning is lemon tea with ginger.*

LIFESTYLE

AVOID: sudden, strenuous physical exertion.
RECOMMENDED: always eat sufficient food, so that you feel full after a meal. This type benefits from hot showers and moderate sunbathing, as well as gentle activities and movement.

THERAPIES

If low blood pressure is accompanied by dizziness, Tibetan doctors use the golden needle or golden hammer therapy.

Menopause problems

DISTURBED BODY ENERGIES: *rlung, mkhrispa*
DISTURBED ELEMENTS: wind, fire
These are *rlung* complaints arising from

the body's hormonal readjustment. Tibetan women hardly ever suffer from menopause problems, and there is no particular mention of it in the *rGyudbzhi*. Most people who live close to nature are unaffected by the phenomenon of menopause problems.

DIETARY RECOMMENDATIONS

Datsen tea (*see page 100*) is helpful for treating menstruation problems as well as symptoms of the menopause. It can be obtained by mail order.

Sinusitis (chronic)

DISTURBED BODY ENERGY: usually *badkan*.
DISTURBED ELEMENTS: water, air.
Many people have chronically blocked sinuses without knowing it. They suffer from the classic symptoms of sinusitis: a continual dull feeling in the forehead, blocked nose and difficulty breathing, but without actually having a cold. Tibetan doctors believe this complaint is linked to a disturbance in the digestive system.

DIETARY RECOMMENDATIONS

AVOID: garlic, onions, radish, sweet things, bananas.
REDUCE CONSUMPTION OF: cold foods, anything frozen, soft drinks from the fridge, sour foods, fats, potatoes, cabbage, milk products.

LIFESTYLE

RECOMMENDED: keep warm, don't expose yourself to wind, after showering always dress immediately in warm clothes. Avoid constipation, as it will make the symptoms worse. People who have the *mkhrispa* or *badkan* constitution types are advised to fast regularly.

THERAPY

Tibetan medicine has a ready-mixed snuff-powder to treat sinusitis, called 'Wangpo Kunsel' (ask a Tibetan doctor). The powder is simply breathed in through the nostrils.

Tibetan herb pills good for this complaint are 'Gurkyung', 'Gurgum 13', 'Dorab', 'Agar 35', 'Nila' or 'Tsenten 18'. The doctor will recommend one of these pills, which can only be obtained on prescription, according to the patient's energy type.

Stomach cramps

DISTURBED BODY ENERGY: *rlung* or *mkhrispa*.
DISTURBED ELEMENTS: air or fire.
In Europeans, pains or cramp-type stomach complaints are usually caused by an infection of the stomach lining (gastritis), stomach ulcers or intestinal infections. Amongst Tibetans, however, a much more common cause of this complaint is dietary. Many Tibetan refugees suffer from stomach pains after emigrating to India. The different climate there requires an urgent change in their dietary habits, but in many cases refugeees are unaware of it. In Tibet, for example, it is common practice to eat dried meat that has been stored for a long time, but in India this presents a grave risk to health.

DIETARY RECOMMENDATIONS

AVOID: any food that is too hot or cold, milk products, cold water.
RECOMMENDED: drinking well-boiled, lukewarm water, particularly when *rlung* or *badkan* energy is disturbed.

LIFESTYLE

AVOID: lifting anything heavy, moving too much, stressing the body through too much activity, showering when you are in pain.
RECOMMENDED: lying flat on your back and relaxing.

THERAPY

SPINAL MASSAGE: Tibetan doctors believe that stomach pains are connected with the large blood vessels below the navel. In such cases, the patient can feel as though they are about to have diarrhoea, sweat a lot and feel weak. To ascertain whether spinal massage will help, measure the distance between the navel and left and right nipples. If these two measurements are different, spinal massage will bring relief. The patient should have an empty stomach, and the masseur should possess some knowledge of massage.

The patient should be seated, with both feet on the ground, and a warm cloth tied around the navel region, with their head hanging downwards. Massage their spine from above, working downwards, for ten minutes. Afterwards, they should eat something.

If the cramps are localized in the stomach region or on the right side, a hot stone or water bottle placed on the spot is helpful.

Upset stomach, indigestion

DISTURBED BODY ENERGY: too little *badkan*; also *mkhrispa*, *rlung*
DISTURBED ELEMENTS: earth, water, fire, air. Indigestion is usually a chronic problem that causes severe discomfort. Sufferers feel heavy after eating, sometimes even sick, and they often experience diarrhoea,

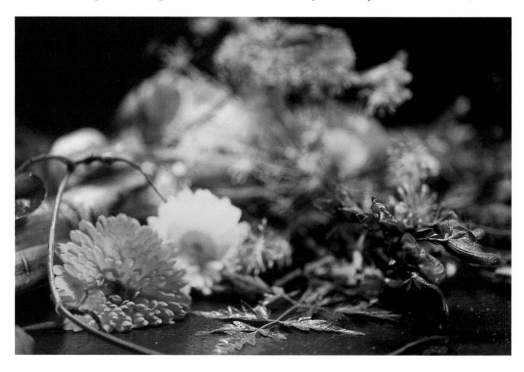

constipation or flatulence. In this disorder the three body energies are not working together, and thus engender too little digestive heat. There is too little *badkan* energy available, while *rlung* brings additional cold into the intestine.

DIETARY RECOMMENDATIONS

AVOID: all mouldy food, uncooked or insufficiently cooked food, irregular eating, eating too much.

REDUCE CONSUMPTION OF: fats, cold milk.

RECOMMENDED: if the complaint is not too severe, fasting will help. Drink plenty of boiled water with salt. Good foods for chronic stomach problems are fish, game, wine, porridge with ginger, and a little lamb.

For less severe complaints, the following tea is helpful:

1 teaspoon pomegranate seeds
½ teaspoon long-grain pepper
½ teaspoon black pepper
½ teaspoon ginger

Mix all ingredients and grind them in a mortar. A teaspoon of this is sufficient for a cup of tea.

If the upset stomach is due to eating raw vegetables, a nettle soup is helpful. Tibetans add the leaves of the Tibetan vine (clematis) to this soup. Take care: the medicinal forest vine is rarely found in Europe. The climbing variety of clematis in our gardens is a cultivated plant, and not suitable for medicinal purposes.

If you have drunk any bad water, add some salt to a glass of water and drink. It also helps to drink a cup of your own mid-stream morning urine each morning. Pour away the first stream and the third stream.

If the indigestion is caused by milk products, boil buttermilk and drink only the liquid from this.

If it is due to bad fat, get some oxidized calcite stone, grind some and drink no more than half a teaspoon dissolved in boiled water.

If your stomach has responded badly to plant oil, drink a teaspoon of lentil flour dissolved in a cup of boiled water.

LIFESTYLE

AVOID: sleeping during the day or exposing yourself to cold wind.

RECOMMENDED: light, not too strenuous jogging.

Physical exercises in a warm room.

TAKE CARE: If metabolic disorders accompany stomach pains, do not do any physical exercises.

Spices as remedies

This list provides a handy reference of the spices that are good for particular complaints. Just increase your consumption of the relevant ones.

SESAME: warming, encourages hair growth, strengthens the body, counteracts *rlung* disorders, increases *badkan* and *mkhrispa*.

MUSTARD SEED: heavy and oily, counteracts *rlung* disorders, promotes sexual and *badkan* energy. Don't use if suffering from constipation or dysuria (painful urination).

ONION: increases bodily heat, supports digestion, improves appetite, promotes good sleep, diminishes *rlung* and *badkan*, good for worm infestation.

GARLIC: of hot taste and sharp active force. Improves sleep and appetite, good for haemorrhoids, skin problems, asthma. Increases *mkhrispa*.

SMALL CARDAMOM: of bitter and hot taste and lightly warming active force. Improves kidney heat, good for excessive urge to urinate and all cold illnesses.

LARGE CARDAMOM: of hot taste and sharp active force. Good for all 'cold' disorders of the stomach and spleen, and improves digestive heat.

NUTMEG: of hot taste and warming with an oily active force. Recommended for heart problems, strengthens bodily and digestive heat, and improves appetite. Good for *rlung* disharmonies.

CLOVES: of hot and bitter taste, of warming and harsh active force. Regarded as a heart tonic, it improves heat in the stomach and liver, and helps with anorexia and indigestion. Alleviates toothache. Good for cold *rlung* disorders.

WHITE CUMIN: of sweet and slightly hot taste, and of oily and also warming active force. Increases bodily heat, promotes digestion, improves the appetite. Good for pneumonia, chronic bronchitis and *badkan* disorders.

BLACK CUMIN: of sweet, slightly hot taste. Good for stomach and chronic liver problems.

CORIANDER: of hot, sweet and salty taste. Good for stomach ulcers, stomach cramps, indigestion, anorexia and severe thirst during infections or fever.

BLACK PEPPER: of hot taste and sharp as well as warming active force. Promotes bodily heat, improves the appetite. Good

for *badkan* disorders, but too much has a bad effect on *rlung* and *mkhrispa*.

LONG-GRAIN PEPPER: when fresh it has a sweet taste, and cooling and heavy active force, increasing *badkan*. When dried it has a hot taste. Improves digestive heat and is good for chronic illnesses and asthma.

GINGER: of hot, astringent and sweet taste, and of dry, warming, light and oily active force. Increases bodily heat, improves appetite, helps with chronic stomach and liver problems, and also diarrhoea, and has an expectorant effect.

ASAFOETIDA: of hot and bitter taste and warming active force. Good for worm infestation and heart problems. Strengthens digestion, decreases *badkan* and *rlung*, strengthens *mkhrispa*.

TURMERIC: of hot and slightly bitter taste. Good for food poisoning and haemorrhoids.

SICHUAN PEPPER: of hot taste. Good for indigestion, stomach cramps, worm infestation and skin complaints. Expands the blood vessels and is good for *rlung* imbalance in the heart.

CARAWAY SEEDS: of hot taste, good for fever accompanied by a *rlung* imbalance. Good for *badkan* disorders and anorexia.

CINNAMON: of sweet taste. Strengthens bodily heat, effective against diarrhoea. Good for lung infections and chronic stomach illnesses.

SAFFRON: of cooling and heavy active force. Good for all liver disease.

LINSEED: of sweet and bitter taste and of warming active force. Decreases *rlung* and increases *badkan* and *mkhrispa*. Linseed paste counteracts swelling.

Healthy recipes from Tibetan cuisine

Tibetans eat very simple and nutritious food. Their main sources of energy are barley and butter. At home in Tibet they need to withstand the cold, but in exile many Tibetans have continued to eat the foods they are used to.

The prime food: tsampa

Tsampa – flour ground from roasted barley – is one of the Tibetans' staple foods. This grain grows even in the climatically extreme conditions of the Tibetan plateaux, and forms the basis of a large number of different dishes.

MAKING *tsampa*

Wash barleycorn and leave it to soften in water overnight. The following day, the water is poured away and the grains spread on a cloth to dry. Once it is more or less dry, roast the barley in a large frying pan and then grind into flour.

Tsampa flour is added to yoghurt or soups, and also Tibetan (barley) beer and the famous Tibetan butter tea. Roasted barley is sweet in taste and has a harsh and light active force. *Tsampa* is a remedy against cold illnesses and *rlung* disorders.

Tsampa SOUP

  9 cups stock from lamb meat and bones
  330g cooked lamb
  1 large radish root
  220g vegetables
  300g tsampa

Put the stock and meat in a pot, slice the radish and vegetables finely and boil until the vegetables are soft. Add the *tsampa*, stirring well. You can enhance this very thick soup with a little butter and a pinch of salt.

Tsampa PORRIDGE

  3 cups water
  1 pinch salt
  a little butter
  400g tsampa

Boil the water and add the salt and butter then stir in the *tsampa*. The porridge this makes is a basic staple for Tibetan children and adults, and is called 'semgong'.

Tsampa BEER

  1 bottle beer
  4 teaspoons grated cheese
  a little butter
  1 pinch sugar
  6 dessertspoons tsampa

Boil the beer together with the cheese, butter and sugar for a few minutes, then add the *tsampa*, stirring constantly, and leave the whole mixture to simmer for a further 20 minutes. Stir every now and then to ensure it does not stick or burn. This beer soup is called 'Kolden' in Tibetan, and is recommended by Tibetan doctors for insomnia, anxiety and depression.

NETTLE SOUP WITH *tsampa*

  400-600g fresh stinging nettle leaves
  2 large pinches freshly ground black pepper
  9-10 cups meat stock
  3½ cups tsampa
  a little salt

Wash the nettle leaves then add them with the pepper to the meat stock and boil for 20 minutes. Stirring vigorously, pour in the *tsampa* and spice with salt and pepper.

Tibetan butter tea

Bhö-cha, Tibet's national drink, is currently arousing interest in the West. In translation the name simply means 'Tibetan tea'. You cannot visit a Tibetan house without being served butter tea. The famous or infamous speciality of *bhö-cha* is its salty-sweet taste and the fact that it contains copious butter, though rumours that this is rancid are not true – it is supposed to be fresh. Butter tea is an extremely 'healthy' drink for the cold regions of the Himalayas – very nutritious, warming and fortifying. The monks value butter tea, both as a welcome break in their long hours of *pujas*, and also as a food substitute. There are Tibetans who drink up to 30 cups a day, very much against the advice of their doctors. Sooner or later, a pulse diagnosis will ascertain that they have high blood pressure. High blood pressure and raised cholesterol levels are classic symptoms found in Tibetans who over-indulge in butter tea. Since this tea is listed here under the heading of 'medicinal diet', we should emphasize once more that butter tea is not suitable for people with high blood pressure and high cholesterol. People with low blood pressure, however, will benefit from *bhö-cha*.

INGREDIENTS:

5g Tibetan tea bricks
(equivalent to 1 dessertspoon black tea)
1 litre water
50g fresh butter
1/5 litre whole-fat milk
1 large pinch salt

Bring the tea and water to the boil and let it simmer for up to 15 minutes. The longer it boils, the stronger the tea will taste but the stimulative effect will be lessened. Pour away the tea leaves and add the buttermilk and salt. Now comes the most important part of the process – the 'plunging' of the tea, for which Tibetans use a *dogmo*, a tube that is closed at the bottom. The *dogmo* can be up to a metre long and 10 centimetres in diameter. The tea is forced up and down with a plunger, which makes a loud gurgling noise (which is why Tibetans sometimes also call the *dogmo* a 'gur-gur'). Since it is unlikely that we in the UK will possess a butter-tea tube, we could follow the example of Tibetans living in the West and simply use an electric mixer.

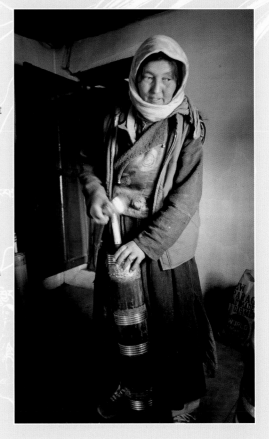

Nettle soup was formerly placed at the entrance to yogis' caves, when they had withdrawn to meditate. It is very nourishing and it also cleanses the blood.

Tsampa WITH BUTTER TEA

1 handful tsampa

1 cup butter tea (see recipe, page 98)

Simply stir the *tsampa* into the butter tea, adding butter to taste, and drink immediately.

Tibetan teas

Drinking tea is one of the Tibetans' favourite occupations. If butter tea is not recommended on health grounds, then they take black or green tea of all varieties, prepared with milk, sugar and aromatic spices such as ginger, cardamom or cinnamon.

There are also medical remedy teas made from Himalayan herbs. Some of the following kinds are available in Europe:

Sorig – a healing brew

'Sorig Tibetan Herbal Tea' comes straight from the pharmaceutical research and development section of the Tibetan Medical and Astrological Institute in Dharamsala. It is the first and only standardized Tibetan tea made by Tibetans and exported to Europe (for mail order, *see page 157*). In translation 'Sorig' means 'knowledge of healing'. The recipe is secret, but it is a herb tea with a very broad spectrum of use, which is perfectly balanced and without any side-effects. It can be drunk by anyone at any time of day, and in any quantities. It is said to be particularly good for colds, coughs and flu, as well as other *rlung* complaints such as asthma, loss of appetite and flatulence. To prepare, add 1 teaspoon of the herb mixture to 1 cup water. Let it brew for 5 minutes then strain.

The four herb teas of Dr Shak

Dr Kalsang Shak is a traditional Tibetan doctor who is also trained in Western and Asiatic medicine. He has a naturopathic practice at Baar, near Zurich, in Switzerland. Years ago, he developed Tibetan herb tea mixtures in an attempt to make Tibetan medicine better known in Europe. To begin with, only the small circle of his patients, friends and relatives were able to enjoy the benefits of the teas, but they became so popular that Dr Shak decided to produce and sell them in large quantities. He joined forces with Padma Limited, a Tibetan company producing Tibetan remedies (*see page 151*), and now Dr Kalsang Shak's teas can be obtained in selected chemists and pharmacies under the name 'Padma – Tibetan Tea'.

'Tashi-Delek'

'Tashi-Delek' is a Tibetan greeting and, roughly translated, means 'May you be blessed with good fortune and well-being'. Based on the teaching of the three body energies and five elements, this tea mixture activates the regulatory capacity of *rlung*, *mkhrispa* and *badkan* energies. The tea promotes the body's own healing forces, brings the energies into balance once more and harmonizes body and spirit. Tashi-Delek tea is a drink for every occasion – even during the day at work – for it has a lightly invigorating effect. Because of its stimulative effect on the metabolism and excretory organs, Dr Shak recommends this as a cleansing tea. It is a mixture of many ingredients, which include ginger, liquorice, nettle, cardamom, pomegranate seeds and peppermint.

'Datsen'

'Datsen' is the Tibetan name for the monthly cycle. This tea is good for treating menstruation problems as well as symptoms of the menopause. It is particularly helpful for alleviating the mood swings many women experience during hormonal changes. Amongst Dr Shak's female patients, this tea's refreshing taste

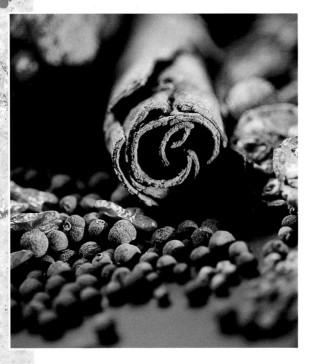

has made it a favourite. It contains, among other things, ground asparagus root, dandelion root, cranberries, turmeric, saffron and cinnamon.

'Gönka'

According to the Tibetans, a healthy immune system is based on spiritual harmony, good digestion and the undisturbed formation of 'Dhang', the subtle quintessence of nutrition. In winter our defences are particularly vulnerable because it is the time of the *badkan* principle, to which are assigned properties such as heavy, cool, damp, dull and oily. The herbal ingredients of this winter tea are intended to reduce the cold badkan energy and bring warmth to the body. It can also be drunk at other times of year to prevent colds, particularly for those with a tendency to *badkan* complaints. The recipe includes rosehips, lemon peel, ginger and cloves.

'Metö'

'Metö' means 'fire of life'. This lightly spiced herbal mixture works chiefly on the digestion. According to Tibetan medicine, a healthy digestive system (the Tibetans say 'a good digestive heat') is a prerequisite for a healthy life. 'Metö' tea is a blessing, especially after a heavy meal. Ingredients include pomegranate seeds, long pepper and ginger.

Incense sticks for healing

Incense is a part of Tibetan medicine, and it works in a similar way to aromatherapy. On inhaling essential plant oils, aromatic fragrances pass through the nose into the limbic system of the mid-brain, the 'seat' of our feelings. This explains the very direct effect of fragrance on mind, soul and our entire sense of well-being.

In contrast to the heavy, sometimes synthetic fragrances of Indian incense sticks, Tibetan incense exudes a light, earthy aroma. There are a number of very good compounds available, but the two most important ones are called Agar 31 and Golar 25. The names refer to the formulae or the chief ingredients contained in them, while the figures refer to the number of ingredients. These products are not always sold under their formula name, but the designation Agar 31 or Golar 25 is usually to be found somewhere on the packet. (For sources, *see page 155*.)

Golar 25

A renowned Tibetan doctor called Geshe Tenzin Pendsok created this incense compound. It is a mixture intended for spiritual rituals, not directly for healing purposes. Nevertheless, Golar 25 contains many medicinal ingredients, including substances to strengthen the heart and inner organs. The effect on the mind and spirit is caused by the fragrant aromas that harmonize body, soul and spirit via the sense organs, thus calming disturbing emotions such as rage, anger or depression. The substances contained in Golar 25, however, mainly emanate a strongly cleansing and clarifying energy. This energy can be used to purify rooms before meditating. The Tibetans use Golar 25 during religious rituals or healing meditations. In the prayer halls of temples and monasteries, its smoke rises as an offering to the highly developed helper beings, called divine energies, who prefer to float in this fragrant atmosphere.

Agar 31

This incense stick is the only one with an explicitly medicinal effect. It gives out very little aroma but is said to be highly effective. The name refers to the agar tree that grows in southern India, whose wood contains essential oils. Agar wood essence not only has a balancing effect on the inner organs but also calms the nervous system and sense organs. Tibetan doctors prescribe Agar 31 for all *rlung* disorders; and it is known as an excellent remedy for altitude sickness, which commonly affects Westerners in the Himalayas.

Rlung disorders that respond very well to Agar 31 include stress-related symptoms such as restlessness, nervousness, insomnia, tension in the shoulders, anxiety, depression, mental imbalance or explosions of rage. 'Agar brings you back to the earth,' say Tibetans. The incense sticks should be used according to need – that is, whenever you feel very stressed and tense.

The best time of day for Agar 31 is in the evening, shortly before going to bed; the worst time is the morning, because the relaxing effect can make you feel sleepy. Leave the windows shut when you burn the incense. You can either simply leave Agar 31 to burn down, or directly inhale the smoke – but in this case only for 5 minutes.

MODERN PHYSICAL EXERCISES BASED ON TIBETAN MEDICINE

Increasing numbers of Westerners are developing an interest in the mind exercises, meditations and physical practices of Buddhism. In their original form some of these exercises, which are over 2,000 years old, are almost impossible for us to follow or grasp. In more recent times, though, some Tibetan doctors and lamas have introduced changes of technique to make these exercises more accessible, and more suited to our needs. Even if fundamentalists complain that the 'new' methods dilute Tibetan teachings, they seem to work extremely well for people both in Europe and in the United States. The systems introduced here are still closely related to their original Tibetan forms.

Tibetan healing yoga Kum Nye

The Kum Nye (*kum nyay*) system of exercises is still relatively unknown in Europe. In its present form it was first devised by the Tibetan lama Tarthang Tulku Rinpoche, who emigrated to the US in 1969, founding the Buddhist Nyngima Institute in Berkeley, California. Tarthang Tulku developed several hundred exercises for his Western pupils, which can easily be performed by young and old without special lessons. His version of Kum Nye is taught in the USA and Europe.

The aim of all the exercises is to harmonize the flow of subtle body energy in the channels (*tsa*) and centres (chakras) of the body, and to free energy blockages. Similar basic ideas are found in Indian yoga, the Chinese Tai Chi and Qi Gong, and Japanese Shiatsu.

The spiritual roots of Kum Nye healing yoga are very ancient. Spiritual body exercises are mentioned in the Tibetan medicine texts of the *Four Tantras*, and in the *Vinaya*, the traditional Buddhist scriptures. The third root of Kum Nye lies in the Tibetan yoga of subtle body energies, known as the *Nying-thig tsa-lung*.

In Tibetan monasteries, Kum Nye was formerly a kind of introduction to further consciousness-enhancing physical exercises. The medicine lamas practised it in order to develop attentiveness and awareness. In its present form Kum Nye can be described as a Buddhist awareness meditation through movement.

The exercises work on a purely physical level as well as on emotional and spiritual planes. Physically they relax muscular tensions. The emotional level becomes apparent when, during practice, suppressed feelings, experiences and memories resurface from the muscles, where they have lain trapped and dormant. When this happens, it is possible to work through the feelings and experiences and release them. With further practice, there is less emotional turbulence to emerge, and you develop more ease. At this point the spiritual dimension comes into its own.

The most important thing about Kum Nye is a kind of internal awareness.

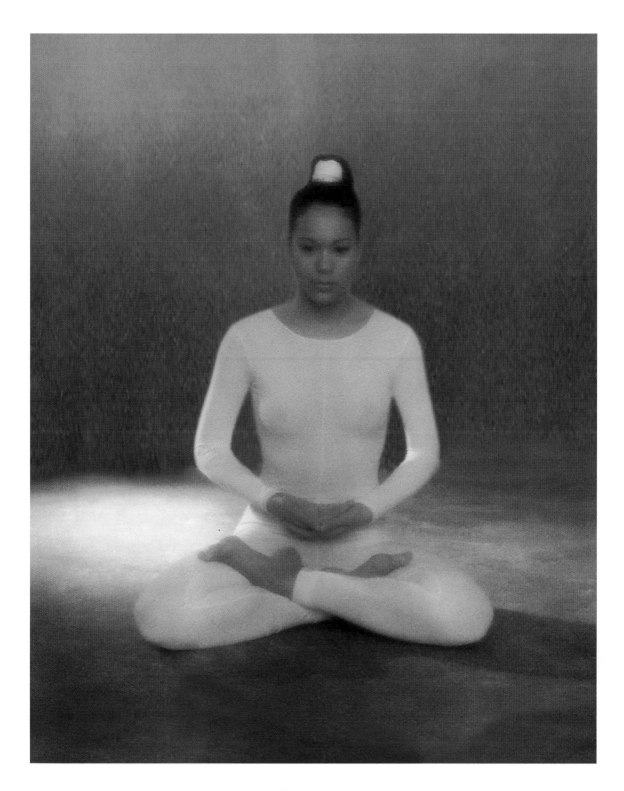

Without this spiritual attitude, all the exercises remain mere technique. Kum Nye is intended to produce awareness and help the participant to develop neutral, objective perception while still remaining actively involved. This kind of awareness is referred to in some texts as wakefulness, inner attention or as bearing witness. It is not a condition that is easy for Westerners to attain: the body is completely relaxed, the mind is 'empty', in other words free of thoughts, and the entire attention is directed to the present moment. All senses are involved in this condition of 'open concentration'. Participants perceive all their physical sensations without judging them. Their attention is lightly directed to their breathing, which should flow through nose and mouth simultaneously during all exercises. Gentle, unforced breathing with a relaxed stomach is important. As soon as any thoughts, judgements or comparisons

surface, you should redirect attention to what is happening physically.

German Kum Nye teacher Matthias Steurich summarized the aim of these exercises: 'Whoever manages to concentrate on the experience of the moment as he does these exercises, is richly rewarded: he gains a sense that undreamed wealth lies in quite simple, daily situations. Kum Nye helps us realize that a more satisfying life need not be sought elsewhere. It is a question of experiencing the moment with all one's senses.'

The exercises are very simple. They do not need to be performed 'correctly' in technical terms. In Kum Nye you learn to perceive more subtly and intensely, expanding the dimensions of experience. Over time these exercises allow us to experience nuances of feeling which we would normally hardly be aware of in our hectic daily lives.

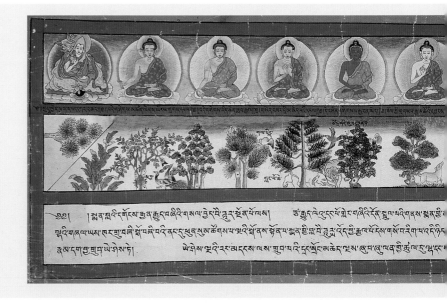

Before starting:

• Prepare yourself to emphasize slowness as you perform the exercises. Always pay close attention to the feelings aroused in you, for they are of crucial importance. Accept them, even if they cause you pain. Pleasant sensations should flow into all parts of your body.

• Always use a meditation cushion or bench for your Kum Nye exercises. This will not only let you relax more easily but also help you to avoid the back and hip problems that can occur during meditation.

• At the end of every session it is important to take time to experience the subtle physical sensations that arose as you tensed and relaxed your muscles. Enjoy the lingering feelings. This kind of perception is an essential part of learning Kum Nye.

• It is important to integrate Kum Nye into your daily life. It is better to practise for ten minutes every day than for two hours once a month. The best thing is to practise Kum Nye each morning and evening.

If you haven't tried Kum Nye before, you should choose two or three of the first seven exercises and practise them until they have become as natural to you as breathing. That could take up to three months. You can vary the sequence if you like. Next, add one or two more exercises and gradually build up your personal programme from there.

'Let your body lead you to the exercises. If you don't have any experience of them, be gentle with yourself and do not try to do too much. Always remember that the quality of movement is of greatest importance, and not the quantity.'

Tarthang Tulku in:
Self-healing through Relaxation

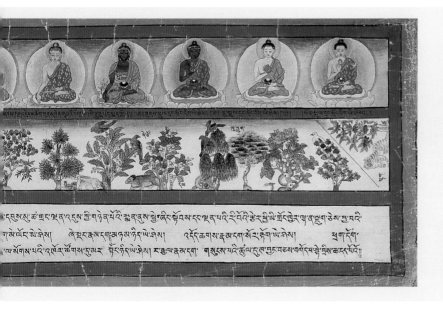

1 The seven gestures

Kum Nye begins with a meditation position. To do it correctly, you should observe the following seven points or gestures. First gesture: sit upright and relaxed with crossed legs. The pelvis should be higher than the legs. It is not necessary to adopt the full lotus position, with ankles laid on the upper thighs. Second gesture: rest your hands comfortably on your knees, with palms facing downwards. Shoulders and arms should be completely relaxed. Third gesture: make sure that your spine is straight but not rigid, so that energy can flow from the base upwards. Fourth gesture: gently pull back your chin. As you do this, your forehead will automatically tilt forwards a little. Fifth gesture: keep your eyes half open and let them rest on a point on the floor, roughly in line with your nose. Your gaze should be soft and compassionate. Imagine that you are a mother lovingly watching her child. Sixth gesture: open your mouth slightly and allow the jaw to relax downwards a little. Seventh gesture: touch the tip of your tongue to the gum behind your upper incisors and feel the curves.

2 Peaceful breathing

For this exercise, you should adopt the postion of the seven gestures described above. Now consciously relax your throat, stomach and spine and breathe gently through your mouth and nose. If you sense tensions anywhere, focus your breath into these places. Your inner dialogue and thoughts should flow into your breath and grow calm.

The breath becomes more and more peaceful until it is completely soft and gentle and flows by itself. If a sensation arises anywhere in the body simply allow it to continue, and observe it. Sometimes it will vanish from one place and reappear elsewhere. Perform this exercise in the morning; during the day, try to become aware of your breathing every now and then.

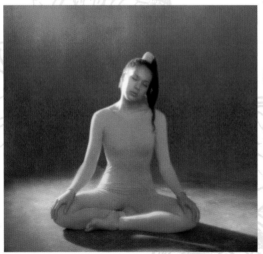

3 Lifting your thoughts

Physically this exercise relaxes neck and shoulders; at a spiritual level it loosens and releases the rigidity of fixed thought patterns. Take particular care to make your movements slow and regular, breathing slowly through mouth and nose, for otherwise you may start feeling dizzy or unwell. Don't try this exercise if you are pregnant or have a neck injury.

Adopt the position of the seven gestures and shut your eyes. Now let your chin sink slowly to your chest. Lift it upwards again until it is pointing towards the ceiling. Consciously and slowly repeat this movement several times. Next, tilt your head to the side. First the right ear tilts towards the right shoulder, then the left towards the left shoulder. Repeat these exercises several times, very slowly. Now, keeping your eyes shut, circle your head slowly in a clockwise direction. Your shoulders should not move, and the circles your head makes should be as large and complete as you can comfortably manage without exertion. If you encounter painful tensions, move your head very slowly forwards and then just as slowly backwards again, so that the muscles can relax and extend. Allow any thoughts to surface. Slow the circling of your head until it almost ceases, and at the same time sense your whole body. Now focus particular attention on the point where the head connects with the spine. Feel an energy there, and then let this travel down the spine and spread out through your whole body, and even beyond it. The head should complete between three and nine circles. Then repeat the exercise in the other direction. Afterwards remain quietly in the seven gestures position for ten minutes, allowing feelings and energy to continue spreading and expanding.

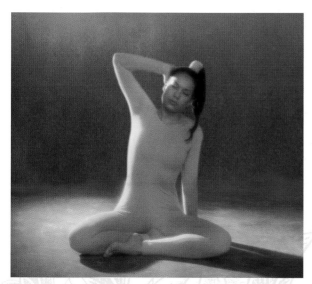

4 Opening your heart

Sit cross-legged on the floor, place your right hand on the floor at a comfortable distance from your body and rest your weight upon it. Place your left hand on your head above the left ear. Your elbow should point upwards. Bend slowly towards the outstretched right arm, forming a great curve with the left side of your body. Your knees should stay as low as possible. The area between ribs and hips is stretched, as are the arm muscles. Hold this position for a few minutes and keep breathing gently. Then allow a full minute to return to the first position. Be aware of the feelings that have arisen in you. Then perform the exercise on the other side, with your left hand resting on the floor, right hand by the right ear and so forth. Perform each stretch between three and nine times. Finally, sit still for a few minutes and let your feelings and sensations resonate.

5 Om ah hum

Sitting in the seven gestures position, breathe gently through your mouth and nose, and think of the mantra *om ah hum*. Imagine the syllable *om* in the upper part of your head, *ah* in the throat, and *hum* in the heart. Now slowly recite this mantra. Quietly say *om* and feel your hands resting on your knees. Now lift your hands, palms upwards, to the height of your stomach, laying the fingers of the right hand on top of those of the left. The tips of the thumbs should touch. Now chant the syllable *ah*. Next place the hands, with palms still upwards, on your knees, and quietly chant *hum*. To begin a new cycle, turn the palms downwards again, lay them on your knees and chant *om*. You should complete a total of 27 cycles in this way, allowing breath, chanting and movement to become one. Afterwards remain sitting for a while.

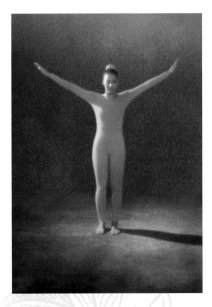

6 Flying

This exercise stimulates your heart and calms your thinking. Stand with your back straight and arms hanging by your sides; your feet should be 10 centimetres apart. Now lift your arms very slowly from your sides, until they are pointing vertically upwards. The backs of your hands should almost touch and the fingers should be stretched. Now shut your eyes and feel your way into your body. The upper thighs should be relaxed and the spine should not curve backwards. After no more than a minute, let your arms sink downwards again. The most important thing is to be aware of all the nuances of feeling and sensation as you make these movements. Allow the energy to flow into your heart. At the next, very slow, lifting of your arms, for which you should also allow a minute, try to let your energy flow outwards from your heart, through your fingers, into the outer world. When your arms are in the air, lightly stretch them. This stretching clears and calms thinking. The arms should be lifted and lowered between three and nine times. You can allow up to two minutes for each raising and sinking motion. After this exercise go into a sitting posture and experience the flow of energy.

7 Freeing up your self-image

This exercise can bring about changes in your thinking and sense of yourself. It also stimulates blood circulation in your skin. Stand upright and cross your arms in front of your chest with the right arm over the left. Hold your shoulders with your hands, keeping your elbows pointing downwards. Now move your right leg over your left and place the right foot beside the left on the ground (*see below left*). In this position, bend downwards very slowly as far as is possible without exertion (*see below*). The head should hang loosely down. Then rise upwards again slowly, bend backwards a little and direct your attention to your feet. Repeat this movement between three and nine times, depending on your constitution, then do the same on the other side with the arm and leg positions reversed. Observe the feelings that arise in you as a result of reversing arms and legs. Then adopt the sitting posture once more and let your sensations resonate.

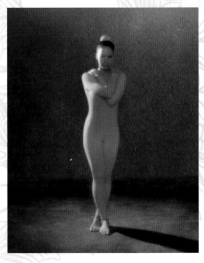

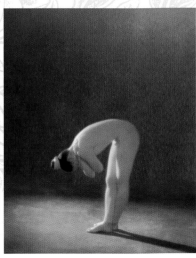

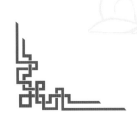

8 *Transforming emotions*

This exercise can help you to transform negative emotions such as anger or anxiety. The energy of the emotions is used to sustain inner equilibrium, and to let more pure energy flow through the body. At the same time the body is energized and the production of hormones stimulated. Stand with your back straight and feet close together. Cross your arms in front of your chest and hold your shoulders with your hands, elbows pointing downwards. Now, keeping your back straight, bend your knees slowly and lower your pelvis as though you were going to sit down on a chair. Your legs should remain together, heels on the ground.

Try to keep your balance without tensing up. At some point or other, tension will prevent you from lowering yourself any further. (Perhaps your heels will lift from the ground.) Be persistent, sense the place where the tension is coming from and resolve it. Then continue your downwards motion, but without actually squatting. Your aim is to reach a particular point, where you sense a particular energy. Try to discover this point – through moving slowly up and down. Once you have found it you will sense warmth, and perhaps a trembling

and a pressure in your knees, too. Remain in this position for as long as you can manage – up to 5 minutes. Pull your chin in a little. Concentrate on the energy in your spine, and observe the tensions that destabilize you. Breathe into these blocked places, even if you feel pain there. Then slowly raise yourself into the upright position again, and stand still for a few minutes with your arms hanging loosely by your sides.

The exercise should be repeated twice – with the same pause between each repetition. Finally, adopt the sitting position again for 10 to 15 minutes, and enter into your inner equilibrium.

Try to sense the feelings and emotions that have arisen in you, and allow them to resonate further. If you remain in this position for long enough, you will eventually feel pure energy flowing through your body. In this exercise you should pay particular attention to the inner tensions that disturb your balance. Even if an emotion is so strong that the tension it causes is painful, breathe into the pain until the tension eases and you sense renewed energy.

Consider the images and memories that had made you tense and try to dissolve these feelings.

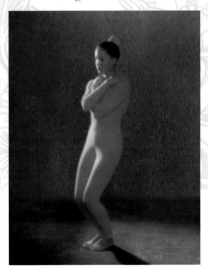

9 Stimulating healing energy

Stand with your feet a little apart and squat on your
toes and the balls of your feet. Form your hands
into fists, and place the first and second knuckles
on the ground in front of you, with your thumbs flat
and pointing towards each other (*see below left*).
Now let your head sink downwards in slow motion.
At the same time lift your buttocks upwards – but
only as far as you can manage without exertion.
Your heels should sink to the floor as you do this.
Now look upwards and remain in this position (*see
below right*). Breathe gently through your mouth
and nose, and be aware of your feelings.

Then lower your head again, and bring your
buttocks back into the squatting position, standing
on your toes and the balls of your feet, with heels
raised, as you did at the beginning of the exercise.
Finally, adopt the sitting position and allow the
feelings that have arisen to expand beyond the
body. You should repeat the exercise twice more.
After each repetition sit down for a short while.
At the very end adopt the sitting position for 10
minutes.

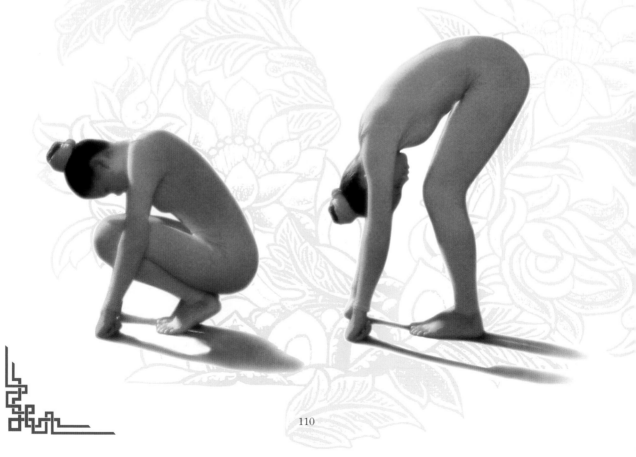

Gyu.lam.Dol
exercises for the subtle energy field

In translation, GYU.LAM.DOL means 'complete liberation from karmic obstacles on the path of development'. These are very simple exercises which primarily affect the subtle energy body. Their aim is to free blocked energies and thus harmonize mind, emotions and body. The strength gained from this promotes spiritual development as well as physical well-being, improving the quality of life.

Swiss Buddhist Antonia Yeshe Dechen Strub-Tusch developed the GYU.LAM.DOL method, based on Tibetan methods of healing. These exercises have a positive effect on ordinary, everyday problems, as well as on psychosomatic and chronic ailments. Strub has been practising traditional Tibetan medicine near Zurich for many years. One of the spiritual teachers who has guided her, lama Thubten Zopa Rinpoche, encouraged her to found a centre for Tibetan healing and gave it the name 'Healing Jewel of the Medicine Buddha's Compassion'. This practice centre for traditional Tibetan medicine (see page 157 for the address) is a meeting place for healthy and sick people who seek physical and spiritual healing through Tibetan Buddhist philosophy and medical teachings. Strub is involved in spiritual-psychological counselling in crisis situations, and health and diet counselling according to the teaching of the three energies, as well as meditation practice and subtle body healing work. She works with groups of

Aids patients and tends those who are dying, as well as their relatives. Above all, she tries to help her Buddhist and non-Buddhist patients and pupils learn to trust their own forces of self-healing.

Antonia Strub teaches people to discover the healing forces in their own hands, and to use this to help themselves and others. Buddhist principles teach that we should all take responsibility for ourselves and that we have the ability to maintain our own health and improve the quality of our lives. 'There is nothing you cannot try to improve through GYU.LAM.DOL,' says Strub, 'for we are working at the subtle energy level, where information is exchanged between mind and body as energies. You can regenerate the energy and information contained in each cell.' Emotions are misdirected or blocked energies that tend to be expressed in negative feelings such as anger, rage, despondency, anxiety, obstinacy, over-excitement or depression. Such emotional states affect our whole physical and mental well-being. GYU.LAM.DOL exercises can dissolve these energy blockages.

From a Tibetan point of view, most problems of the civilized world derive from an imbalance of *rlung* energy. Typical symptoms are nervous disorders of heart, circulation, stomach and intestine, as well as anxiety and sleeplessness, allergies or dystonia. 'People with *rlung* disorders are often haphazard, chaotic, and unfocused, and tend to try to do too many things at once. Or they never stop saying how well they are feeling. But inwardly they are completely out of balance and feel

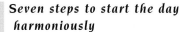

wretched.' GYU.LAM.DOL teaches us to know our inner difficulties and our positive qualities. The exercises help us on the path of evolution and liberation from all conflicts. They teach us to recognize true, deep feelings, and to distinguish them from emotions. This spiritual, energy-purifying process occurs in a gentle, harmonious way, and is often unnoticed. Occasionally people practising these exercises realize with surprise that they no longer get upset about things that used to send them into a frenzy. If you can't change your circumstances, the wise thing to do is change your attitude to them instead.

Seven steps to start the day harmoniously

The following exercise, consisting of seven steps, should be performed the moment you wake up, while still lying in bed. The trance-like state when you waken is the best time to strengthen mind and body energies for the day ahead. The whole exercise takes about 20 minutes. Maintain the individual hand positions without pressure until you feel a pleasant prickling sensation at these points. Sometimes you may have to take a deep involuntary breath – a good sign that a tension has dissolved.

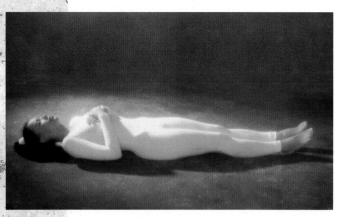

1 Cross both hands over the heart chakra: the left hand should lie under the right in the middle of the breastbone. This position opens and strengthens heart vibration energy, promoting love and compassion, trust and inner calm. You can also do this exercise during the day – for instance, when you need to make decisions that require both heart and head.

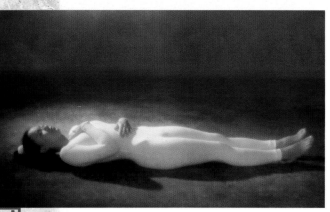

2 Place the right hand lightly on the throat chakra: the thumb and middle finger should rest slightly above the collar bone. The left hand rests on the solar plexus, with the thumb touching the end of the breastbone. This position has a harmonizing effect on breath and speech and it gives the organs of metabolism and digestion the best preparation for assimilating and digesting food.

3 Place your right hand at the base of your skull: wrist and middle finger should be touching its edge. The left hand lies on the navel chakra, about the breadth of two fingers below the navel. The thumb touches the navel. This exercise clears the head, releases energies in the body blocked by aggression, and promotes inner calm and strength. It thus enables you to begin the day with mental clarity.

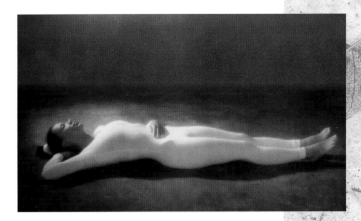

4 Place your right hand very lightly on the crown chakra, at the top of the head. The fingers of your left hand should touch the root chakra – that is, the pubic bone. This releases tensions in the nerve tissue and muscle tone. All energies in the body and the aura around it are harmonized. Overall this step promotes physical and mental well-being.

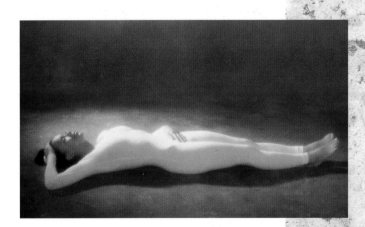

5 With your left hand still resting on the root chakra, move the right down to the heart chakra. Now breathe deeply in and out a few times. In this position the body's upper and lower energy circulations are balanced.

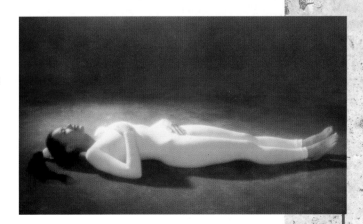

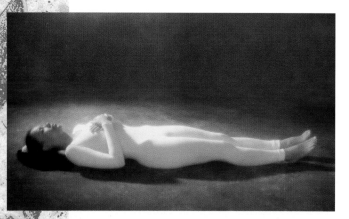

6 Place your left hand once more beneath the right on top of the heart chakra – as in step 1 – to bring the exercise to a harmonious close. This strengthens the heart, which is then better able to affect your thinking and reason.

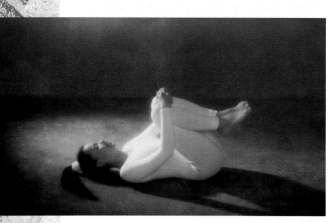

7 Remove your hands very gently from the heart chakra position. Before you get up, stretch once lengthways and then hug your knees in your arms (*see left*). Breathe in deeply through the nose and out again through the mouth and as you exhale press your knees lightly against your chest. This exercise stretches the whole spine and releases blocked energy. At the same time it stimulates the intestinal tract and makes it ready for evacuation.

Finger exercises to balance rlung energy

Important nerves linked to the brain end in the fingertips. The seven finger exercises described here enable you to reach the nerve tissues via the brain, so that blocked energies can be released. In this way, it is possible to gain control over powerful mood swings as well as the typical *rlung* disharmonies mentioned earlier. Perform these exercises whenever you can withdraw for a while – or just before an important conversation, during your lunch-break, in the bus, during a train journey or in the midst of daily activity. Do them sitting or standing, or even lying down, if you are ill and unable to get up, for instance. They can be performed either one after another or individually, as you need. Bear in mind the aim of each exercise as you are doing them. If a particular finger position enhances confidence, for example, concentrate on this theme: visualize a situation in which you have experienced confidence. Sense and enjoy this feeling. Relax and breathe deeply. The better you can focus inwardly on the aim of the exercise, the more clearly you will experience its effect. With time, your ability to control negative emotions will increase.

114

1 With your palms facing upwards, place your left hand on top of the right with the thumbs just touching. This connection promotes mental and physical stability and clears the mind. It counteracts depression and low spirits and harmonizes all three bodily energies.

2 Touch the tips of your index fingers with the tips of your thumbs. This promotes self-confidence, lessens anxiety and harmonizes *rlung*. It is a good exercise to perform before exams or important conversations.

3 Touch the tips of your middle fingers with the tips of your thumbs. This connection promotes vitality and creative forces. It lessens aggression, releases blocked energies and harmonizes *mkhrispa*. If there is anger in the air and the blood is rising to your head, perform this finger exercise and breathe deeply.

4 Touch the tips of your ring fingers with the tips of your thumbs. This promotes emotional clarity and releases pressure, harmonizing *badkan*. This is an exercise for staying focused in the present moment. It is good for people who tend to drift back into the past, and then grumble about it and can't let it go.

5 Touch the tips of your little fingers with the tips of your thumbs. This helps you to appear as you truly are, and lessens psychological stress, harmonizing *rlung*. In this way it helps you to reconcile your inner needs with external circumstances. Anyone who pretends something he does not actually feel lives in a fragmented world. This position helps people to experience themselves authentically and to convey an accurate image.

6 Clasp your hands and let them rest in your lap. This exercise stabilizes your overall condition and lessens intolerance. It rounds off the sequence of exercises and indicates the conclusion of a whole. For instance, you can lay your hands in your lap like this at the end of the day or after completing some work. This harmonizes upper and lower energy circulations.

7 Hold your thumbs in your fist. This exercise harmonizes the two sides of the brain, earths and calms you after mental over-exertion. It is also good for helping you fall asleep, as it stabilizes the mind and emotions.

115

Exercise for positive strength

This is good for low blood pressure, regenerating and energizing the whole body, for staying awake, and for whenever you are required to be creative. Lie on your back on the floor, with legs loosely outstretched. Rest both hands in your groin, with your middle and ring fingers in the base of the groin. Lie in this position until you sense warmth beneath your hands.

Holding the calves

This position helps if you have too many thoughts racing through your head in the evening, if your 'mental wires' are glowing red hot, or your body is too hot, so that you can't fall asleep; it is even good for sunburn. Sit down, bend forwards and cross your arms, holding your calves in your hands for 10 to 20 minutes. This will draw energy from the head downwards. For over-stimulated, hyperactive children who cannot fall asleep, calf-holding is done as follows: sit down at the foot of the bed where the child is lying and simply take his calves in your hands. Sit quietly and do not speak.

Exercise for a harmonious end to the day

In order to reflect on what has happened during the day, and to prepare your metabolism for the night, adopt the following position in bed before falling asleep. Lie on one side and slightly bend the leg that is uppermost. Lay the lower hand on the uppermost shoulder, so that your fingers touch the shoulder muscle. The fingertips of the uppermost hand should touch the back of the right thigh (*see below left*). This position promotes deep, refreshing sleep.

Tibetan meditation exercises

Meditations are some of the most important spiritual remedies in Tibetan medicine. They directly counteract the three spiritual poisons of greed, hate and blindness, which according to Tibetan and Buddhist perspectives are the cause of all suffering – whether physical illness or mental and emotional problems. For the spiritually orientated Tibetan, meditation is a normal part of his religious life and serves him as a kind of mental hygiene to keep the spirit healthy. The following meditation exercises were specially chosen for Westerners. They are 'visualization' meditations.

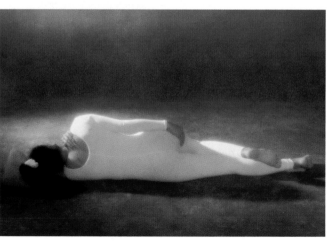

The meditation posture of the Vairocana Buddha

Spirit and body are dependent on each other. While actual meditation involves the mind and spirit, the body needs to adopt a position which encourages rather than hinders mental processes. The seven-step meditation posture of the Vairocana Buddha is regarded as a perfect stance for meditation:

1 The eyes shouldn't be either wide open or completely closed. The gaze should be directed downwards along the line of the nose.

2 The head should bend slightly forwards – rather like a full ear of corn on a straight stalk. Nose and navel are in vertical alignment with each other.

3 Teeth and lips rest in their natural position and are not pressed together. The tip of the tongue lightly touches the gum behind the upper teeth. This position limits the flow of saliva so that you do not need to swallow so often during meditation. The breath flows calmly and naturally. Don't artificially slow it down or force it.

4 The shoulders are straight and at equal height. Arms and shoulders are relaxed.

5 The back is straight and upright, without bending too far backwards or forwards.

6 The hands rest in one another in your lap, palms turned upwards. Both hands are slightly curved so that the tips of the thumbs touch one another and form a triangle.

7 The legs are crossed in a full or half lotus. In the full lotus each foot rests on the upper thigh of the opposite leg, with the sole pointing upwards. The half lotus is easier: the left foot rests on the floor under the right leg and the right foot lies on the left upper thigh (or the other way round).

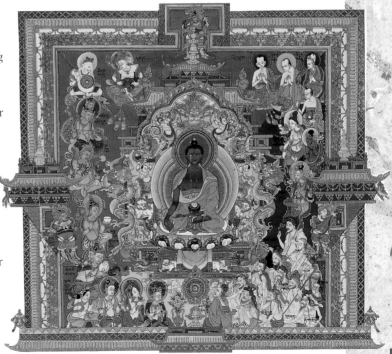

The White Light meditation

This meditation comes from the Tibetan Buddhist text LAM.RIM – 'stages on the path to enlightenment'.

Choose a comfortable position – it could be the meditation posture described above, or you can lie down or sit on a chair. It is important for you to be able to relax and direct your full attention to the meditation, and to positive motivation and attitude to life. Ask yourself: 'What is the sense and purpose of my life?'

The answer is: the sense and purpose of my life is not only to solve my own problems and find happiness for myself. Since I can perceive that every feeling creature experiences suffering and moments when the spirit is obscured, the purpose of my life is to liberate all sensate beings from their problems and the cause – the obscuring of the spirit – and lead them to initial and then ultimate happiness, which is the everlasting, greatest happiness of perfect peace. This is the sense and purpose of my life.

The foundation of my life is not small and narrow but as great as endless space. I have the responsibility and also the potential to liberate all sensate beings from their problems and obscurities and help them towards happiness, in particular the ultimate joy of full enlightenment. In order to be able to carry out this great service for all sensate beings, I wish to develop wisdom and the right methods, such as loving kindness and compassion towards all creatures. To do this I desire strength and long life. To attain all this I will carry out the White Light meditation.

The meditation

Inhale deeply and slowly then exhale. As you breathe out, imagine that all your illnesses, all disturbances from other beings, from unconsidered actions and thoughts, and the impressions these have left in your consciousness, are being cleansed. They should all evaporate from your body like dirty black smoke and dissolve into nothing. As you breathe in again, imagine that strong, white rays of light are radiating outwards from the heart of the Buddha, who symbolizes the perfect pure spirit of full enlightenment. You can imagine a different image, but it must be something that for you embodies love, compassion, wisdom and healing. This clear, white light completely floods and illuminates your body and cleanses you from all sickness, from all disturbance by other beings, unconsidered actions and thoughts and their impressions in your consciousness. Feel how your body assumes the nature of the white light. All suffering vanishes, body and spirit are freed. From the top of your head to the soles of your feet you are filled with great joy and happiness.

After you have experienced this joy, imagine that your life has been lengthened and that your positive energies, which are the cause of your happiness and success, have increased. Wisdom and compassion have unfolded within you, as has your understanding of the path to liberation. During the visualizing and sensing of the white light you held your breath for a short while. Now rest in this joyful state while breathing again. When you feel that the time has come, repeat the exercise.

The Heart-Fire-Giving-and-Taking meditation

This visualization meditation was specially conceived by Antonia Strub as a warm-up to the subsequent classical TONG.LEN meditation. Recall a deep love you had for another person, and allow the warming feeling of this memory to grow within your heart. Sense the tingling and warmth in your heart. Let this warmth flow. Send it to the person closest to you at the moment, and sense how this person is nourished and warmed by it. This in turn allows the warmth, strength and love in your heart to grow further. Now your heart fire is so great that you can send it further – to a large circle of people in your environment. The hearts of these people will be touched by it: they sense strength, joy and tingling in their own hearts, their heart fire is kindled. Now all their sufferings and problems can melt in your heart fire and flow away. Now imagine that you take up these molten sufferings as fuel for your own heart fire. Thus it is continually fuelled and continues to grow. From your heart fire, rays of loving kindness, warmth and compassion flow in all directions; and all creatures receive these benevolent rays. The heart fire of these creatures is fed and all their sufferings dissolve and flow away. This healing circulation of giving and taking opens your heart for loving kindness and compassion, and connects you with all your fellow human beings.

Traditional TONG.LEN meditation

This visualization exercise is a meditation to counteract viruses, illnesses and emotional disturbance. It has a very profound effect. Those who practise it honestly and correctly can attain very positive results. Rato Chubar Rinpoche developed it for an HIV-positive pupil. After you have completed your usual, preparatory prayers, chant the following invocation. It does not matter whether you recite it in Tibetan or English as long as you understand and feel what you are saying.

INVOCATION

de na tsun lama tuk je chen
ma gyur dro wa dig drib duk ngel kun
ma lu dan da dan la min pa dang
da gi da shen la tang wa yi
dro kun da dank den par jin shi lo

'May the seeds of all unvirtuous actions,
all hindrances, and the sufferings of all living beings now ripen in me,
and, as I offer up all my happiness and my virtues,
may I be blessed with the power to give joy to all living beings.'

MEDITATION

I imagine my viruses, my sickness, my self-centred and negative emotions, attitudes and actions, as a black sphere in my heart. Then I imagine all living creatures from the six realms of existence (people, animals, 'hunger spirits', devil beings, gods and demi-gods) gathered around me in human form – particularly those who are burdened by the same sufferings as I am. I think of their sufferings, of the suffering of all those who are sick as I am, or who bear the seed of this suffering within them, and of all the sufferings of the other realms of existence.

Now I imagine drawing all the suffering out of these beings, in the form of a black ray of light from their right nostrils; and letting it flow into my left nostril. This black ray of light flows directly down into the black sphere in my heart and completely destroys it. I imagine that I have wholly freed all these beings from their sufferings.

I pray that my suffering may take the place of theirs; and I imagine that this black sphere of my viruses, my sickness and my self-centred and negative attitudes, has been destroyed. Then I imagine giving all my happiness, my wealth and my positive energy to all living beings. All this streams from my right nostril, in the form of a white ray of light, into all these beings, and fills them with happiness and positive energy.

(Copyright for the GYU.LAM.DOL methods and meditations: Antonia Yeshe Dechen Strub-Tusch)

TIBETAN MASSAGE AND ACUPRESSURE

A true massage culture, as exists in Japan or Thailand, never developed in Tibet. One of the reasons for this, no doubt, is the climate. In winter, the best time for massage, sub-zero temperatures prevail in Tibet and undressing is a dangerous pastime. Social and religious factors also play a role. The Tibetans seldom massage the whole body but only certain regions of it.

Nevertheless Tibetan massage is regarded as a very effective external therapy, which supports other treatment methods.

The doctors themselves only massage in exceptional cases, for strictly medical purposes. Massage for relaxation or mild indisposition belongs to the tradition of folk medicine, and is carried out by relatives or close friends. Within families it is usually the women who pass on their knowledge to one another. At least as important as the techniques employed are the massage oils or ointments, which Tibetans believe 'bind the wind' – that is, balance excess *rlung* energy. Massage ointments, often enhanced with spices, are very easy to make (*see page 127 for some recipes*).

In the ancient medicine texts, massage is regarded as a 'hot' remedy, and thus recommended against 'cold' illnesses, in particular classic *rlung* disorders, but also against combined *rlung/badkan* cold-type illnesses. It is used for all nervous, stress-related and psychosomatic ailments and tensions, including joint and menstruation problems, tinnitus and nervous need to urinate. Lobsang Rapgay, a Tibetan doctor who now lives and teaches in California, broadened the massage instructions in the *rGyudbzhi* to include the acupressure points of Japanese shiatsu, and recommends his techniques, described below, as an accompanying therapy for anxiety and depression.

Tibetan massage, which is broadly similar to these techniques, should be carried out on a regular basis. In the winter Dr Rapgay recommends three sessions a week. In the summer the body needs less energy-input from other sources, so massage is best used only for specific medical treatments. The best place for a Tibetan massage is lying on a mat on the floor; the best surroundings are a warm, peaceful room not too brightly lit; and the best time of day is the late evening or before midday.

Those giving a massage should ensure that the partner they are going to massage is relaxed. Ask your partner to take a few deep breaths, spread some massage oil or butter on your palms and begin.

Stroking

Every massage begins with long, stroking movements, which distribute the massage oil or butter over the body in the following sequence: head, ears, palms, soles of the feet, chest, back, arms, legs. Stroke with light, even pressure – rather as a mother would stroke her child's head. Stroking not only stimulates skin function but also relaxes the body and prepares it for the massage to follow.

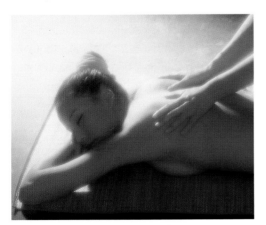

Rubbing

Now make wide, strong, circular movements with the balls of the thumbs or the whole palm. It is important not to exert any pressure. Use this technique to treat all tense places, in particular stiff joints. Avoid the sensitive zones around the eyes, the heart and the genitals. Rubbing improves

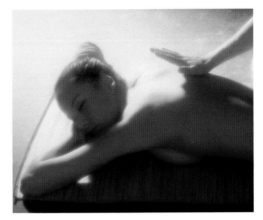

circulation, makes the muscles more flexible and relaxes the whole shoulder, neck and back area. Try to proceed intuitively, and address the places that need attention. If the person being massaged has cold hands or feet, pay particular attention to them. In the stomach region, make sure you perform the circular motions in a clockwise direction.

Kneading

You should use different parts of the hand for kneading, depending on which areas of the body are being massaged. For arms and hands use your thumb, index and middle finger; and for large areas of musculature – that is, all fleshy areas such as thighs and buttocks, the soles of the feet, hands and shoulders – use your

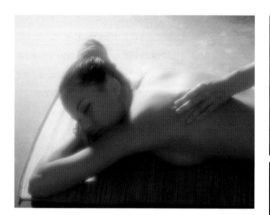

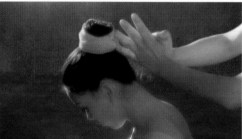

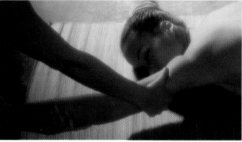

whole palm with all the fingers. Begin with the shoulders and continue with the arms, upper thighs, back, buttocks and calves. The muscles should become pliable like dough. The chief purpose of kneading is to loosen tension and 'soften up' hard areas. Tibetans know that tension building up through stress and suppressed emotion accumulates especially in the fleshy parts of the body. Ensure that you keep the movements even, and take care around the joints if the person being massaged has complaints such as arthritis. Always avoid causing pain.

Pulling and tapping

Pulling is used for the arms and legs, not the torso. Lightly pull the fingers, moving along their length up to the tips, without causing pain. Do the same thing with toes and then the arm (*see above right*), which is pulled with the whole hand as if you were trying to lengthen it from the shoulder. Take care to perform these pulling movements slowly and gently. The legs are gently pulled lengthways.

Tapping is used only on the head and must be done very lightly. Clasp your

hands and stretch out your fingers then tap your fingertips very carefully on the skull, starting from the middle of the head and radiating outwards in all directions (*see above*). This tapping activates brain function and enhances concentration. Ask the person you are treating whether he finds this pleasant. Tapping too hard can give people headaches.

Pressing and circling: acupressure

Acupressure is not mentioned in ancient Tibetan medical texts, but it forms part of modern Tibetan massage. This technique probably arrived in Tibet via China and Japan. For everyday purposes Tibetans only use 10 different acupressure points, while specialists employ 25 to 36. These points are pressed deeply and circled with the thumb for a minute each in small clockwise movements. Three turns of a circle are used for small children, and very old or weak people. For relaxation

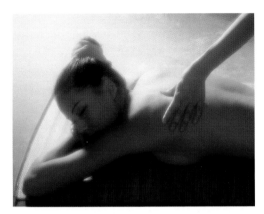

massage, and for healthy people or those with only minor ailments, each point is circled 25 times; but only 5 circles are used for pregnant women and extremely sensitive patients. There are different circumstances where the points are massaged either 3, 7, or 21 times.

The most important acupressure points

Only the 11 most important acupressure points are listed here:
• Front fontanel: this can be found the breadth of 12 fingers upwards from the tip of the nose.
• Top of the head (vertex): the highest point of the head, about 20 finger breadths upwards from the tip of the nose. There is a small hollow in the fontanel, which is the softest point on the skull. This is also where the golden needle is inserted in 'golden needle therapy' (see page 50).
• Small (rear) fontanel: this lies in a small hollow at the back of the head, about 4 four finger breadths behind the vertex of the head.
• Temple points: the temple hollows a little above the cheekbones.

• The point in the middle of the rear of the head, where the skull joins the neck.
• The two horizontal fontanels at the rear of the head: two hollows lying on the right and left of the back of the head, a little above the place where the skull joins the neck.
• The jugular point: the small hollow below the larynx, where the two ends of the collar bone meet.
• The deepest part of the armpits.
• The seventh cervical vertebra: this is the one that stands out most prominently when the head is bent forwards.
• Middle of the palm.
• Middle of the sole of the foot.
You will find descriptions of other points in the following treatment examples.

Massage and acupressure for specific ailments

Tension headaches

Put either a little warm sesame oil or some nutmeg butter (see page 127) on the scalp, and massage the skull strongly with your fingertips and the whole palm. If this doesn't help, bind a cloth firmly round the head for 20 minutes, then remove it and massage the following acupressure points with nutmeg butter: • vertex of head • small fontanel • front fontanel • the two temple points • two further points on the left and right side of the back of the head; these can be found by pressing along a horizontal line at the level of the ears round the back of the head, until you come to a sensitive place where there are small dips in the skull • the neck point in

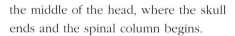

the middle of the head, where the skull ends and the spinal column begins.

Constipation

Tibetan doctors regard constipation as 'descending *rlung* energy', which hinders intestinal function. Warmth is particularly recommended for this ailment, especially in the lower abdomen. The following three acupressure points should be massaged with sesame oil: • the solar plexus • the two points 2.5 centimetres left and right of the navel and • the two points 5 centimetres left and right of the navel.

Anxiety and panic attacks

If fear or panic arises, you should immediately massage the two most important acupressure points: • the hollow beneath the larynx between the two collar bones and • the mid-point on the breastbone that lies equidistant from the two nipples.

If you do not have any massage oil to hand, just use some olive oil – or, if nothing is available, do without. Press and circle the points for a few minutes. Then you can massage the other points, or have them massaged, if possible with warm sesame oil. These points are: • the fifth and • sixth thoracic vertebrae. To find them, start counting from the most prominent cervical vertebra downwards. The prominent vertebrae are the ones which are massaged, the so-called spinous processes. Other acupressure points are: • the vertex point, that is the soft dip at the highest point of the head, and • the two temple hollows.

Insomnia

Before going to sleep you should dribble five drops of warm sesame oil into each ear. After this, prepare some nutmeg and aniseed butter (*see page 127*), or use warm sesame oil as an alternative, and massage the following points: • vertex point of the head • the small fontanel • the front fontanel • the two transverse fontanels at the back of the head • the two temple hollows • the most prominent cervical vertebra • the fifth and sixth vertebrae (*see Anxiety and panic attacks*) • the two points in the middle of the palms and the soles of the feet • the deepest points of each armpit.

Dizziness and tinnitus

Apply warm sesame oil or nutmeg butter to the following points: • the hollows directly behind the earlobes (particularly evident when the mouth is open) • the vertex point of the head • the small fontanel • the front fontanel • the two rear fontanels on either side • the hollow between the collar bones (Charaka point).

Tiredness

Apply either warm sesame oil or nutmeg butter to the whole body, using the rubbing and kneading massage technique (*see page 121*). Afterwards work on the following acupressure points: • the two temple points • the rear transverse fontanel points • the seventh thoracic vertebra • the eighth thoracic vertebra • the ninth thoracic vertebra • the eleventh thoracic vertebra. The first thoracic vertebra is the one after the prominent cervical vertebra.

Tiredness and painful eyes

Prepare some aniseed butter (*see page 127*), or use warm sesame oil. Lie down with your head against the arm or back of a chair. Put some of the massage oil or butter on your fingertips and rub it into your closed eyelids. After this, massage the following acupressure points with the same oil: • the two rear transverse fontanels • the two forehead points 5 centimetres above the middle of the eyebrows • the jugular point (middle of the collar bone) • the seventh cervical vertebra (most prominent vertebra in the neck) • the point in the middle of the rear of the foot, found by tracing a horizontal line backwards from the ankle • the fourth thoracic vertebra • the eleventh thoracic vertebra.

Pains in the lumbar spinal column

Use aniseed butter to work on the following acupressure points: • the upper thigh point • the place on the hips that the middle finger touches when your arm hangs down by your side • the fifth lumbar vertebra (a little below the waist) • the first sacral vertebra 2.5 centimetres below the fifth lumbar vertebra • the second sacral vertebra • the third sacral vertebra • the fourth sacral vertebra • the fifth sacral vertebra (last vertebra before the coccyx). After this, apply aniseed butter to the whole lower part of the back and the legs, then rub and knead these areas. Finally rub lentil flour into the massaged skin and vigorously rub off any remaining oil. After this the person who has been massaged should rest and relax for at least 30 minutes.

Menstruation problems

Here, too, aniseed butter is recommended as a massage oil. Apply it to the rear thigh and loins, and in front to the lower abdomen. Massage these areas with gently circling clockwise movements. Then begin with acupressure massage on the following points: • the two hip points (where the hip bones end at the waist, at the top of the ilium) • the bladder point, two finger breadths below the navel, and one finger breadth left and right of this point • the first lumbar vertebra • the fifth lumbar vertebra • the first to fifth sacral vertebrae (the fifth sacral vertebra is the last one before the coccyx).

Final rub with flour

Every Tibetan massage and acupressure ends with a concluding ritual: rubbing the whole body with flour. This 'rubbing down' has a double effect: firstly it removes any excess oil from the skin; and secondly it gives the body an invigorating rush of energy.

Overall, the concluding rub with flour enhances circulation and improves skin colour. It is done as follows: take about two handfuls of barley or chickpea flour and use it to rub the body in generous stroking movements working downwards. Leave the massaged person to rest for 10 minutes with the flour on his body. When he gets up, the flour should be softly brushed off. Showering is not necessary after this 'rubbing down', for not only does the flour absorb all the excess oil efficiently, but it also has a beneficial skin-cleansing effect.

Making your own Tibetan massage oils and creams

Massage oils and creams have two advantages in Tibetan medicine: firstly they make massaging easier, and secondly they protect the body from getting too cold, by enclosing it in a warm layer of oil or fat. Tibetans have been making their massage creams and oils for centuries, using substances that are readily available in their kitchens. Butter and plant oils form the basis. In former times, animal fats or bone marrow were also used for massage.

Butter

For Tibetans, butter is not only a chief nutrient but also an important remedy used both internally and externally. It belongs to the taste sphere 'sweet', and its warming properties are particularly helpful for *rlung* disorders. For massage purposes, butter is melted and applied while still warm. It is mainly used for tired muscles, weak circulation, stress, tension, anxiety and depression. It is even said that butter has a regenerative effect on the skin. When used in massage, the butter usually has nutmeg, aniseed or barley flour added to it. Butter that has been stored for a while is best for

massage. In ancient medical texts, one-year-old butter is recommended for massage to cure stress symptoms. Yak butter stored for a year is regarded as a remedy for neurosis, and the butter-fat obtained from it is a good remedy for strengthening the memory. Butter-fat, one of the major remedies in ayurvedic medicine, also plays a role in Tibetan medicine. It can simply be used in place of melted butter. To make butter-fat, melt a piece of fresh butter in a pot over a low flame, and spoon off the butter froth forming on the surface. What remains in the pot is 'clarified' butter or butter-fat.

Plant oils

Sesame oil is by far the most important plant-based massage oil. Tibetan medical texts recommend it for use all year round. It is of 'sweet' taste and lightly warming. It gives the body energy, tones the skin and is a proven remedy for stress and over-exertion.

Sandalwood oil and the oil from agar wood (*Aquilaria agallocha*), which are also used, are only suitable at certain times of year.

Agar oil belongs to the 'bitter' taste sphere, and is regarded as a hot substance. It is described as very 'nutritious' and restorative. Its warm properties mean that it is most suitable for winter massage.

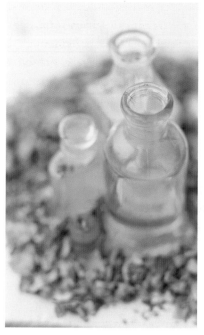

Agar oil relaxes the muscles and nerves and stimulates circulation.

Sandalwood oil is of astringent taste and cooling action. This means it is good for massages in warm seasons. It relaxes the muscles and improves skin tone. Since massage is thought to be harmful at high temperatures, the Indians add sandalwood oil to a cooling footbath during hot periods. Place two dessertspoons of sandalwood oil in a footbath with cold water and bathe the feet in it for 20 minutes. This is a proven remedy for insomnia on hot summer nights.

Tibetan fats

In former times, Tibetans used animal fats for healing wounds

and for massage in certain cases –
for example, for back tensions,
impotence and weak kidneys.
Otter fat was particularly praised
for massaging the back, lower
abdomen and kidneys. Nowadays
these fats are hardly ever used.

Recipes for massage butter

The following recipes are very
simple. Prepare them shortly
before the massage, since the
butter must be warm and fluid.

Nutmeg butter

INGREDIENTS

1 teaspoon grated nutmeg
1 teaspoon barley flour
2 teaspoons melted butter

Mix the melted butter with the
other ingredients, until you get a
paste-like consistency. This
massage cream is good for all
anti-stress massages and for
typical stress symptoms such as
tension headache, insomnia,
dizziness or pounding heart.
VARIATION: *1 teaspoon ground
nutmeg, 1 teaspoon melted butter.*
Mix both until you get a creamy
consistency. This variation is
particularly good for pounding
heart, anxiety, restlessness and
inner tensions.

Ginger butter

INGREDIENTS

1 teaspoon ginger powder
1 teaspoon melted butter

Mix both ingredients to a cream.
The ginger butter can be applied
to relieve pain in large or small
areas. Massage it into the skin.

Aniseed butter

INGREDIENTS

1 teaspoon aniseed powder
*1 teaspoon melted butter (yak
butter is recommended)*
3 dessertspoons chickpea flour

Mix the aniseed and butter until
they are creamy. Tibetan doctors
recommend this mixture for eye
problems and ailments – for

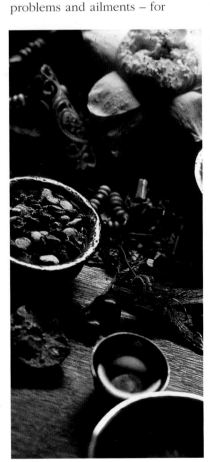

instance, tired or ageing eyes, and
also for eye pains. The eyes
themselves are definitely not
massaged directly, but rather the
soles of the feet. Wash the feet
thoroughly then apply the cream
to the soles, and rub and knead
them. Rub off excess fat carefully
with the chickpea flour, and allow
the feet to rest for a few minutes.
Finally lay two hot stones (but
not too hot) on the soles. If
possible, the stones should have
been heated in a charcoal or
wood fire.

Nutmeg and aniseed butter

INGREDIENTS

1 teaspoon ground nutmeg
1 teaspoon aniseed
1½ teaspoons melted butter

Gring the aniseed in a mortar and
mix the ingredients to a porridge-
like paste. This massage cream is
recommended for anxiety,
depression, insomnia and other
emotion-related ailments.

Musk butter

INGREDIENTS

*1 pinch musk powder (from the
musk plant)*
½ teaspoon melted butter

Mix both together. This makes
a good massage cream to
cure insomnia. Massage the
temples with it before going
to sleep.

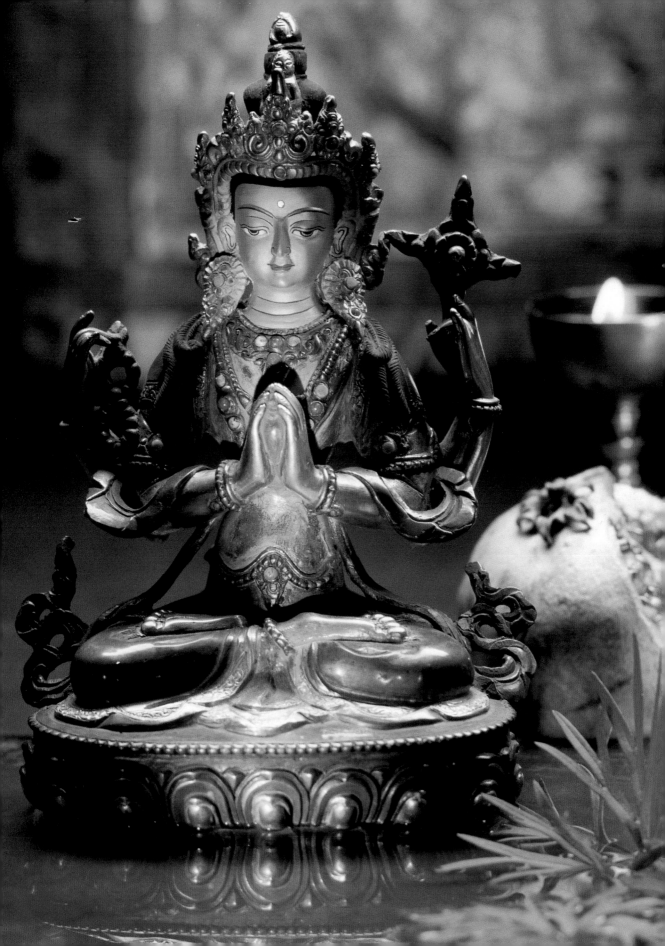

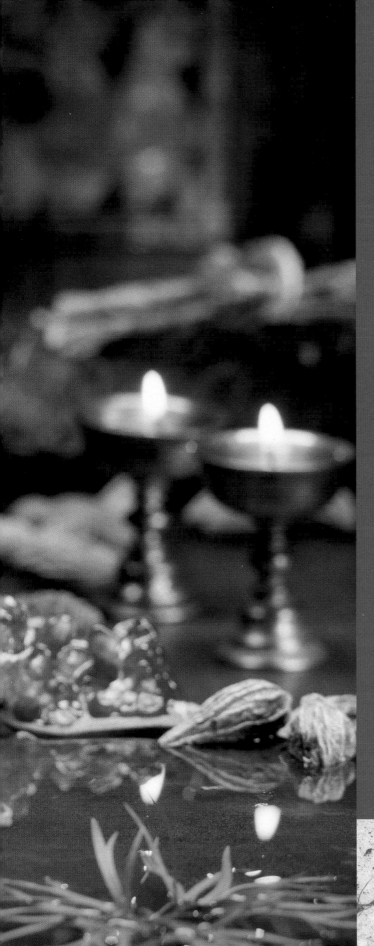

Tibetan Medicine in Asia

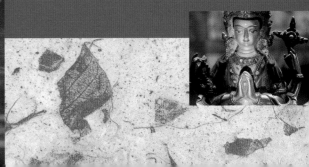

Chapter 4

The Situation in India

There are about 130,000 exiled Tibetans, of whom roughly 100,000 now live in India – and the numbers are increasing all the time. The flow of refugees never dwindles. Every year between 2,000 and 4,000 Tibetans flee their homeland, most of them monks, children and young adults up to the age of 25. But the path to freedom is highly dangerous, for the escape routes lead over mountain passes 5,000 to 6,000 metres high, and many freeze on the way.

In Nepal's capital, Kathmandu, at the southern edge of the Himalayas, exiled Tibetans have set up a reception camp. Here refugees receive any urgent medical attention they require, and meet a representative of the UN refugee commission. After a short stay they continue their journey by bus to Dharamsala in northern India. There, in 'Little Lhasa', the Tibetan government has its headquarters; and here too lives the generally acknowledged political and religious leader of Tibet, the Dalai Lama.

In Dharamsala the refugees enter a hostel where they sleep on plank beds in rooms for 80 people. There they wait for the day when the Dalai Lama will give them an audience and his blessing. For many, this is the high point of their lives. After this they move on again. Children enter care homes or children's villages;

Previous pages: Four-armed Buddha, butter lamps and pomegranate. In the background is a thangka with prayerwheel

young men and women go to boarding schools, where they learn writing, reading, Hindi and English.

The Dalai Lama has gone to great lengths to look after the health and education of his people. It was only two years after his own flight, in 1961, that he founded the Tibetan Medical Centre in Dharamsala.

During the 1960s a network of schools for Tibetan children was established. The Dalai Lama delegated responsibility for these to his sister Jetsun Pema, who is five years younger than him. To cope with the enormous flood of refugee children from Tibet, the 'Tibetan Children's Village' (TCV) was formed, with headquarters in Dharamsala. Nowadays this organization supports ten villages with over 11,000 children and young people, in Tibetan settlements between Ladakh in the north and Bylakupe in the south of India. Some of these children's villages are members of SOS International. The government in exile runs a total of 85 schools, many of which are exemplary boarding schools. Almost all pupils find work after leaving, and 20 per cent go on to universities and colleges, later returning to the settlements as doctors or teachers. There is another conglomeration of Tibetan settlements around the southern Indian town of Mysore. A total of 35,000 exiled Tibetans live there in five settlements, having cleared and cultivated jungle terrain assigned to them by the Indian government. The largest settlement, Bylakuppe, is 50 kilometres from Mysore and has 10,000 inhabitants. Besides a

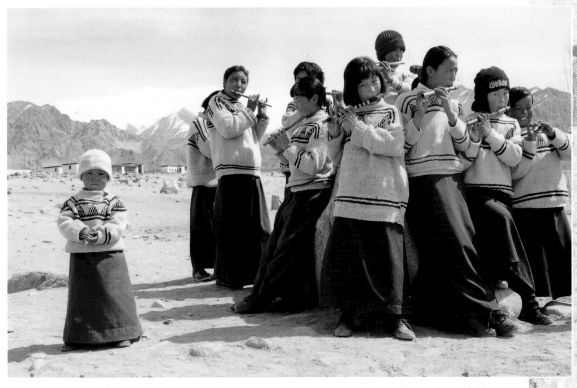

In outstandingly well-run children's villages set up by the government in exile, Tibetan refugee children find a new home. A scene from the SOS children's village at Choglamsar, near Leh.

children's village, the TCV also runs an agricultural project here, in which grains, bananas, mangos and coconut palms are cultivated and livestock are reared.

Even more than in northern India, life in the south is characterized by extreme poverty. Many Tibetans are forced to spend half the year travelling as traders round Indian tourist resorts. The goods they sell are generally made in craft workshop centres that have been set up with the help of international donations. Traditional Tibetan crafts are resurrected here: young Tibetans learn to make knotted Tibetan rugs, paint *thangkas*, manufacture silver jewellery, weave cloth, and sew bags and

traditional costumes, just as their forefathers did.

Around Mysore four large Tibetan monastery centres have been established. They see themselves as outposts of the enormous former 'mother-monasteries' in Tibet, which were largely destroyed during the Cultural Revolution, then rebuilt and now reopened under conditions stipulated by the Chinese. These are the three monastery universities of Gelugpa ('Yellow Caps') Sera, Drepung, and Ganden; and Tashi Lhumpo, the former seat of the Panchen Lama. Many monks living in Tibet choose to flee to the newly built monastery centres in southern India, for they suffer from severe repression in their homeland, and are bereft of all spiritual leadership there.

Like their leader the Dalai Lama, most Tibetans believe in a 1,500-year-old prophecy that predicted their land would one day be occupied but says that it will eventually be liberated again.

The Tibetan Medical and Astrological Institute

The Tibetan Medical and Astrological Institute of His Holiness the Dalai Lama lies on a forested mountain slope halfway between Lower Dharamsala, a valley inhabited by Indians, and Upper Dharamsala, 5 kilometres higher and crowning the peak of the mountain at 1,800 metres above sea-level. McLeod Ganj, as this place is also called, is the 'capital' of exiled Tibetans in India, a small, isolated nest in the mountains with views over the snow-covered southern slopes of the Himalayas, and 13 hours by car from Delhi. It is a village bursting at the seams: as headquarters of the government in exile and the Dalai Lama, 'Little Lhasa' has been drawing people from all over the world for decades. Here you will meet spiritual globetrotters and drug users, as well as Tibetans who have fled over the mountains from their homeland. Buddhists of every shade meet here to attend the Dalai Lama's talks. Journalists report from here on Tibetan affairs. Not least, Dharamsala is also a mecca for all those seeking help from Tibetan medicine. It is not in vain that the government in exile vaunts the

successes of Tibetan medicine on its Internet homepage: 'Its effect on hepatitis is, according to some Westerners, close to a miracle. It also counteracts chronic diseases.'

'Many people who have tried everything else,' says Wilfried Pfeffer, a student of Buddhism in Dharamsala, 'seek help from Tibetan medicine. The consciousness-raising healing process in Tibetan medicine is much more potent than in any other method of healing.'

There are now nearly 40 branches of the Tibetan Medical and Astrological Institute throughout India and Nepal. In Dharamsala, it is constructed like a village, with buildings linked to each other via footpaths, winding steps and squares, surrounded by lovingly cultivated plants. Tseten Dorjee, the public relations guide, takes visitors on a tour of the grounds. All the requirements of Tibetan medical practice are combined here: there is a general surgery with a dispensary; a factory where pills are manufactured; the medical school with a library and an art department (for painting Tibetan medicine pictures); a research and development unit; an astrological institute; a large museum, opened recently in the presence of His Holiness; an administrative department with a mail order section for dispatching herb pills to some 1,400 patients all over the world. There is even a hospital (with two rooms for patients); and, amongst all the other facilities, there are also lodgings for the students and employees. Lady Dr Dachoe earns 4,000 rupees a month – roughly £100 sterling. This 36-year-old doctor, whose name is actually Dawa Choedon, sometimes sees as many as a hundred patients a day in the surgery, so none of them gets a longer consultation than the much-criticized three-minute sessions of Western GPs.

In the waiting room is a throng of people: Tibetans, Europeans, Americans. Some sit on the floor, others stand. There are two counters in the waiting room – one for paying, the other for dispensing medicines. And there is one toilet, into which the doctor periodically disappears with a urine sample. The two treatment rooms are only separated from the reception area by a curtain; and since family members are also admitted to consultations, there are people sitting and standing everywhere.

Dr Dachoe sees patients together with her assistant Dr Sonam Wangmo Khangshar. Both sit at their desks and each of them takes one of the patient's wrists, left or right, to measure the pulse. In this way they can exchange views about the diagnosis. Pulse diagnosis is the most important method of diagnosis used here. Sometimes patients are asked to show their tongues, and sometimes a urine sample is required, but blood pressure is seldom taken. Methods of treatment mainly involve prescriptions for pills and advice about diet and lifestyle, though owing to limited time this is usually just a single sentence. The other consultation room is that of Dr Lobsang Wangyal. He is the second of the Dalai Lama's three personal physicians. He spends some of his time overseas, travelling around giving lectures, taking

pulses and offering medical consultations. The Tibetan Medical and Astrological Institute doctors are constantly receiving invitations to travel abroad like this. During his absence, Wangyal's room is used for special treatments such as cauterizing or moxa therapy, during which mantras are chanted, but these are only carried out on auspicious days.

On the morning I visited, the following cases were dealt with:
• Lobsang, 46 years old, institute employee. Has suffered from digestive problems for a long time. Gets diarrhoea when he eats heavy foods. For the last week he has been taking pills prescribed by Dr Dachoe, and has come back to be monitored. He says he is already feeling better. He is told to keep taking the pills, and not to eat heavy foods, raw foods or cheese. He should eat only freshly cooked food.
• Rinzin Ghado, 49, a nun from the nearby Dolma-Ling monastery. She has kidney problems and swollen feet. The doctor examines her ankles and has her assistant take her pulse. In her book she has noted that the nun has been taking pills for the last six weeks. There is a 25 per cent improvement. She is given a pill prescription for 15 further days, and is told to eat fewer potatoes, and less sweet and salty things.
• An English woman in Tibetan costume enters the room and, instead of a greeting, she stretches out her upraised arms to the doctors: 'Goar 25 is great. I'm feeling much better. I need more of them. And I also wanted to ask you . . .' 'Shhh,' says the

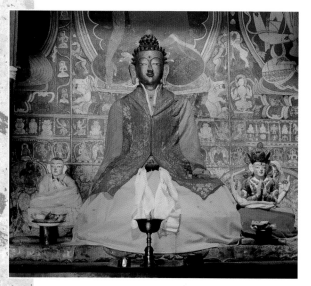

doctor. 'First the pulse, then talk.' The doctor asks how the bleeding is; it's still continuing. 'I will give you a different medicine, Goar 16. It's good for the immune system.' The woman leaves the room happily.

• Londen Peju, 50. It is obvious from her clothing that she doesn't have much money. She complains about dizziness and feeling sick. The diagnosis: low blood pressure, too little *rlung* energy. The last time the woman came here because of arthritis, which has improved. Londen Peju receives free treatment and medicine in the Tibetan Medical and Astrological Institute, because she falls into the category of 'poor'. Medical treatment is free for all those without means, for institute employees and all people over the age of 65. Students, monks and nuns pay half-price. Foreigners from the West pay the most. The following day I had an opportunity to watch Lady Dr Kalchoe Qusar giving cauterization treatment. The patient, a 35-

year-old monk called Dawa Tsering, only recently fled here from Tibet. Before that he was in prison for four years and was tortured by the Chinese. 'Electric shocks,' explains the doctor, who specializes in refugee conditions. The Chinese take electric rods, of the kind that are used in Europe during cattle transportation, and use them as instruments of torture, inserting them into their victims' bodily orifices. The monk still suffers from the consequences of this torture and therefore comes to see the doctor often. 'Complete *rlung* disturbance,' comments Dr Qusar, 'dizziness, depression, headache, great tension in the shoulders and back.' Today he is receiving cauterization treatment. Resigned, the monk closes his eyes as the glowing coin-sized end of the iron touches the top of his head. He doesn't even flinch. The same procedure is repeated at two points behind his ear and on the chest bone. After that a cupping vessel is pressed to his shoulders. 'This helps with his depression,' says Dr Qusar, and taps the hot cup to fix it there. 'In a few days he will feel better.'

Dr Dawa manages the department for producing medicines. A hundred and sixty different preparations are made here. In some cases, the herbs are cleaned, peeled, cut, sieved, sorted and laid out to dry by hand; in others, modern machines grind, pulverize and mix them. This long process usually produces round, brown pills; but sometimes creams and herb powders too. Some types of medicinal powder are swallowed with water, while others are boiled in water and reduced until only one-third of the original liquid remains. These are the decoctions.

When I visited, a powder was being mixed to make 'Men-chik' medicine. The 'hot' active forces of the ingredients warm up digestive heat to counteract cold *badkan* disorders, explained the head of department. I noted down the Tibetan names of the herbs: *se-dru*, *pi-pi-ling*, *shing-tsa*, *sug-mel* and *gur-gum*.

We arrived at the astrological institute, which collaborates closely with the staff who produce the pills. 'Sometimes someone calls me to ask whether it is a good time to process a particular substance,' explains the astrologer Tsering Choezom. She then either gives the go-ahead or advises a different time. It is particularly important to be precise in the case of the precious pills, as there is an optimal moment for each process involved. Sometimes one hour makes all the difference.

The doctors working in the surgery also follow the directions of the astrological section. For instance, some days are unfavourable for 'hot' therapies, such as moxibustion, cauterization or golden needle therapy. And there are times when it is better for the patients themselves not to receive treatment. Tibetan astrology is more orientated to the lunar rhythms than Western astrology, and another difference is that the Tibetan calendar only has 360 days in each year.

Anyone who wants to understand the medical institute better should go there after 5 o'clock one day, when the doctors and employees finish work. Then the large square behind the administrative building becomes a great, private meeting place. Doctors who have just been treating patients arrive carrying their babies on their backs. Children who have been in the institute's crèche all day can come out and play in the open. The 32 doctors employed there live with their families in small two-room flats, next door to their colleagues. A little further away live the 52 students of the medical school. Their lives and futures are dictated by Tibetan medicine.

An international view: Namygal Gusar

Namygal Qusar, 39 years old, belongs to the younger generation of Tibetan doctors who have studied in exile. He was fortunate enough to learn from the great masters of the ancient tradition and collaborate closely with them; but he sees the future of Tibetan medicine as working hand-in-hand with Western methods.

Namygal Qusar knows his Tibetan homeland only from his parents' descriptions. He grew up in a Tibetan settlement in southern India and came to study at Dharamsala in 1981. He was particularly proud to have been a personal pupil of the late doctor Dolmar Lobsang, who ran a renowned practice in Upper Dharamsala. Qusar completed an additional training in pharmacology. Since 1987 he has been working in the research department of the Tibetan Medical and Astrological Institute, and is currently its assistant director. Among other innovations, he developed the new 'Sorig' products, which are now distributed throughout the world, as well as the Tibetan herb teas described in Chapter 3, and the much-praised ointment against eczema (*see page 87*).

Although he is a firm believer in the idea of Tibetan and Western medicine complementing each other, Qusar turned down an offer to work for a Western pharmaceutical company. He prefers to conduct his experiments from a Tibetan viewpoint. For instance, he is managing a project researching the efficacy of Tibetan medicine in treating diabetes; and further researches are planned into using herb pills to treat sinusitis, asthma, cancer and tuberculosis. Just recently he presented his institute with a report on suspected links between drinking-water quality and increased arthritis in the new Tibetan settlement at Karnakata. Qusar had a bacteriological water analysis conducted along modern Western lines, but simultaneously recommended treating the water with an ancient calcite remedy. The Tibetan Medical and Astrological Institute in-house periodical praised this experiment as a 'further example of the efforts of the Research and Development section to analyse the efficacy of Tibetan medicine in prevention and treatment of modern diseases.'

For some time Namygal Qusar has been running his own business. In his Tibetan Herbal House, close to Dharamsala, he manufactures healing incense sticks and develops modern variations of ancient herb pill formulae, along the lines laid down in the *rGyudbzhi*'s ancient medical texts. In future, Qusar will use these pills to treat his own patients. This initiative is welcomed by the Tibetan Medical and Astrological Institute because, in the face of growing numbers of patients from the West, there is starting to be a shortage of pills.

For many years now, Qusar has received invitations to give lectures all over the world and his association with a number of European medical institutes has put him in a good position to adapt his consultations on lifestyle and diet to Western conditions. As just one small example, he explains: 'For certain illnesses Tibetan doctors recommend freshly cooked foods. This refers to the old Tibetan custom of keeping and continually reheating the same food for weeks on end. But in the West people normally eat freshly cooked food anyway, so this advice is superfluous.' In contrast, there are very few Tibetans who grow ill through over-work. Patients in the West, on the other hand, often suffer from exhaustion syndromes, which are hard for a Tibetan doctor to understand. In order to make a correct pulse diagnosis, such a doctor really needs comparable experience.

In future, Qusar plans to spend six months of each year in Europe, so the waiting lists to see him there ought to grow considerably shorter.

The personal physician of His Holiness

Tenzin Choedrak is at present probably the most important master of Tibetan medicine, because the 75-year-old personal physician of the Dalai Lama is one of the few Buddhist monk-doctors still alive who were trained exclusively in the traditional medicine of ancient Tibet.

Tenzin Choedrak was born in 1923 in the Tibetan region of Nyenmo. At the age of 10 he entered the Nyenmo Chö Di Gompa monastery as a novice of the Bodong order. At the age of 17 he was chosen by his monastery to go to Lhasa and study Tibetan medicine at the renowned Chagpori school. He finished his training at the age of 24. While treating patients in the Mentsikhang, the Tibetan state institute and hospital, Choedrak also studied pharmacology. This is the most difficult field of Tibetan medicine, to which only the best pupils are admitted, but Choedrak passed his exams with flying colours and soon became a pharmacologist and later the institute's chief apothecary. Because of his many great accomplishments, he was summoned at the age of 32 to become personal physician to His Holiness the 14th Dalai Lama.

For three years Choedrak pursued this work. But in the fateful year of 1959, his life and that of all Tibetans changed. Twelve days after the flight of the Dalai Lama, Dr Choedrak was arrested, and then incarcerated for the next 21 years. He spent 17 years in prisons, 6 of these doing hard labour in a stone quarry. As an intellectual, Choedrak was labelled a member of the 'reactionary clique', and from the beginning he was appallingly tortured. One of the most humiliating methods was 'thamzing': he was brutally bound to a cross, and fellow prisoners were forced to beat him with heavy shoes, until he would denounce His Holiness. 'In all that occurred there,' he says, 'no blame attaches to my fellow prisoners.' Nothing could bring him to accuse his master, the Dalai Lama. Twenty days later another 'thamzing' was inflicted on him. For half a year the prisoner wore handcuffs and leg irons day and night, to which a heavy iron ball was attached.

Then, as a 'prisoner with incurably reactionary thinking' he was transferred to a prison in China, close to the Gobi desert, and subjected to very hard forced labour, as well as 're-education'. He was given next to nothing to eat. Choedrak chewed leaves that the wind blew within reach. Of his 302 fellow prisoners, 300 died. After three years Choedrak was transferred to the Tibetan prison of Sangyip. There he could perform Tum-mo exercises in secret, and concentrate on chanting mantras, by pretending he was reading Chairman Mao's *Little Red Book.*

Things grew a little better. In the mid-1970s two Chinese officers came to consult him about their health problems. Choedrak felt their pulse 'without any ill will in my heart and without hatred'. The medicines he prescribed helped the officials a good deal. From then on, Choedrak was allowed to leave the prison on Sundays, and on other days he treated patients in the prison. Since many of his patients soon recovered, his case was reviewed by the Chinese authorities. In 1977 Choedrak was released, and in 1980 he moved to India. In Dharamsala he was immediately appointed chief personal physician by the Dalai Lama. Since then Choedrak has lived and worked in the Tibetan Medical and

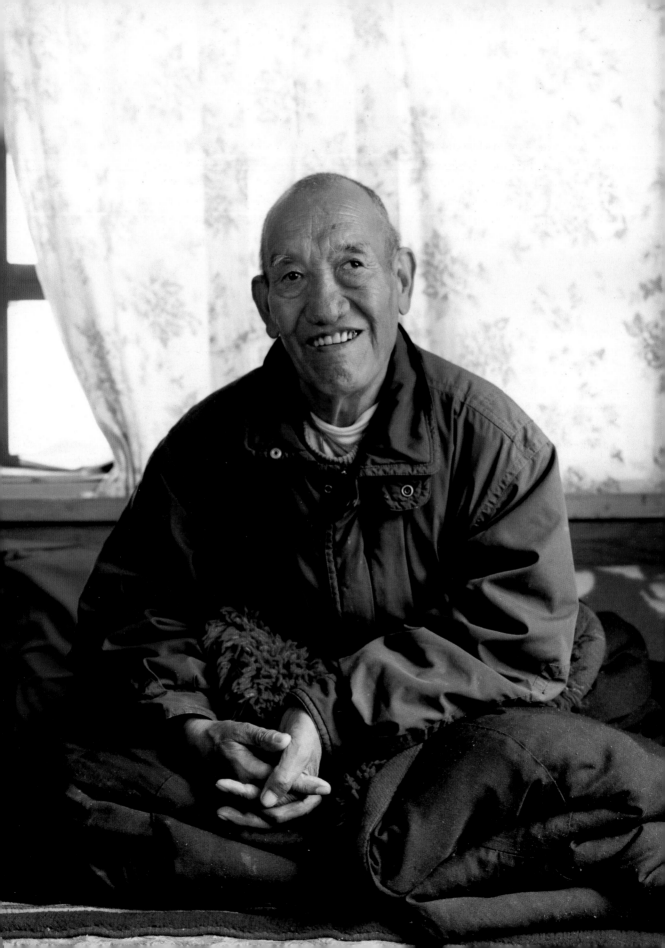

Astrological Institute in Dharamsala, where he holds many positions. He is chief doctor, as well as director of the pharmaceutical, materia medica, and research and development departments. The jewel or precious pills are still manufactured under his guidance.

In 1997 a film about Tibetan medicine was released – *Das Wissen vom Heilen* (*Knowledge of Healing*) by Franz Reichle – and it featured Choedrak in the central role.

Like many great Buddhists, this 'senior doctor' lives very modestly, without possessions. In his humble one-room flat in the Tibetan Medical and Astrological Institute grounds there is a couch, a few books on the shelves and a little crockery. While I was researching this book, I visited him in his flat for a consultation and to ask him some questions.

Choedrak, a delicately built man with a warm gaze, indicated that I should sit down beside him on the couch. Without a word he took my wrist, pressed a little on the pulse and abruptly let my hand fall again. The interpreter said I should rest a little first, for my pulse was not yet clear enough. He asked if I had come by foot.

I replied no, that I especially took a taxi. The regulations stipulate that on the morning of a diagnosis you should avoid physical exertion and drinking coffee. I had also adhered to the rules for the

People come to see Tenzin Choedrak from all over the world. He treats the Dalai Lama, as well as American actor Richard Gere.

evening before – no meat, no alcohol, neither too little nor too much exertion, neither too little nor too much sleep.

After a while Dr Choedrak took my right arm once more and placed the tips of his index, middle and ring fingers on my pulse. His hands were as warm as his gaze, which scrutinized my face. As he put questions to me, he continually altered the pressure of his fingers as though he was playing a stringed instrument. Was I taking any medicines? Yes, a prophylactic preparation for bowels and intestines, and vitamin pills. Had I already taken them today? Yes. Were my monthly periods OK? Yes, no problems. Did I have any digestive problems at present? No, I replied truthfully, not dreaming that I would have that very evening. Dr Choedrak could already tell this from my pulse.

As his fingers continued to press and release at various places, the finest motions of my organs and my soul were revealed to him. He took a brief look at my tongue and then began to chant a mantra in a melodious tone. The interpreter listened attentively and kept nodding her head. Choedrak talked continuously and pressed my pulse. The magic of his hands and voice penetrated my inmost being. I felt completely transparent. Apparently there was much to say about me. The interpreter continued to nod her head – she understood. She told me my organs were basically sound, and all my problems stemmed from the mind. The moment I became mentally tense, my physical ailments grew worse, and I got back pains, stiff bones and digestive problems. That is why I should always do my utmost to be moderate in my thoughts and harness extreme emotions. I should not be too depressed about failures, nor too euphoric about success, nor should I be extreme in my judgement of other people. I should aspire to balance and moderation in all respects, and in diet as well. I should eat a little of everything but not too much of one thing, and less coffee and cheese.

The interpreter kept repeating this theme in various forms, speaking of balance of mind, and disturbances of the life-sustaining *rlung* element, which affects moods and thoughts. As she explained this, Dr Choedrak wrote out a prescription. I should take two kinds of pill: half an hour before breakfast three 'Yuker' pills; and half an hour after supper three 'Duitsi 11' pills. I should chew these first, then swallow them with some lukewarm, boiled water. The morning pill would strengthen my inner organs, such as kidneys, liver and spleen; and the evening pill would help counteract my *rlung* disorders. What *rlung* disorders? I wanted to know. Well, the stiff muscles in my neck and back, stiff joints and lumbar pains. I hadn't actually mentioned these, but I had read that patients tend to be told by the doctor what their ailments are (or are about to be), rather than the other way round.

At the institute's dispensary, 88 light-brown and 86 dark-brown pills were put in white plastic containers and carefully labelled. Pills for a month. I paid 450 rupees for the medicine, and 100 for the consultation, which is the equivalent of less than £10 sterling.

'If your symptoms have gone after a month, it is good,' said the interpreter. 'If not, please send us a photocopy of the prescription and describe your ailments. The letter will be shown to Dr Choedrak, and then we will send you new medicines.'

Interview with Dr Choedrak

It is said that many people in the West suffer from rlung *disorders. Are my ailments therefore typically Western?*

CHOEDRAK: There are no culturally determined differences in illness. Ailments derive from lifestyle, dietary habits and climate, and these can affect everyone. In some regions people eat too many sweet things and get diabetes; others eat too much meat or drink too much alcohol and get problems related to that.

Can you explain why so many Westerners are interested in Tibetan medicine?

At the beginning of the century there was great interest in Western, allopathic medicine. But when it turned out that there were risks and side-effects involved, people started looking everywhere for natural forms of medicine. Tibetan medicine interests people so much because it includes the natural environment and the five elements. The five elements can be rediscovered everywhere in the wide universe, everywhere in nature. Man is also composed of these five elements, as are the herbs and the medicines we make from them. When making medicines we lay

140

great value on the taste spheres and the active forces of substances, as well as their digestion-enhancing effect. By doing this we take account of the five elements. This correlation between Tibetan medicine and the human being means that no side effects come about. Another reason for this is that we have the teaching of the three bodily energies.

Do you believe that Westerners could become good doctors of Tibetan medicine, even if they were not Buddhists?

Tibetan pills have a good healing force. Whether they are effective or not depends on the doctor's motivation and not his beliefs or religion. Tibetan medicine says that there is a karmic connection between the doctor and his patient. When this connection is good, the medicine prescribed by the doctor will be effective. If there is no karmic connection between doctor and patient, the medicine can sometimes be rather ineffective despite the doctor's best efforts.

Does a doctor notice what sort of karmic relationship he has with a patient?

Yes, a doctor notices.

Should a doctor send a patient away if he finds that he has no karmic link with him?

If the doctor has no karmic relationship with the patient, this means that the medicine itself is more important. Ultimately medicines are based on the

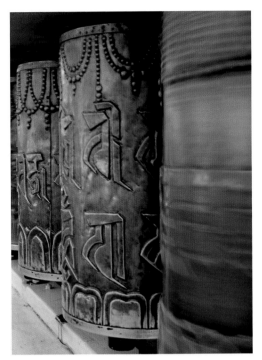

power of the taste spheres, the taste spheres after digestion, and on specific active forces and qualities. These definitely help the patient. But the effect of the medicine on the body is less than the effect of the karmic connection. The medicine will help, but not as much as the karmic connection.

May I ask whether you sensed any karmic connection with me as you took my pulse?

[*Choedrak laughs.*] Why are we sitting here opposite one another and holding this detailed conversation? Why have we met here? Because we have a karmic connection.

Tibetan medicine says that many illnesses are caused by wrong thinking. Can these medical teachings counteract a wrong attitude to life?

Wrong thoughts always arise through a certain mental attitude. These wrong thoughts are the cause, in turn, of unhappiness. One should break this vicious circle by training the mind. There are many ways to do this. This mental training is important, for unhappiness due to false mental attitudes impairs the body, which also of course contains the five elements. The bodily disorders which arise as a result can be cured by medicine. The physical imbalance of the five elements can be re-balanced with pills.

Are disorders caused by wrong mental attitude also common among Tibetans?

Absolutely. It is not true to say that only Westerners have mental disturbances. These exist everywhere in the world. Among Tibetans too, mental imbalance such as sadness and unhappiness have greatly increased. On the other hand there are many good people in the West too, who help the poor, fight for justice and work for better conditions for others.

Dr Choedrak, thank you for this conversation. I am pleased to have met you.

I am pleased that you are interested in Tibetan medicine, that you wish to help others with it, and that you came on a long journey for this purpose. I am also pleased to have met you.

The situation in occupied Tibet

The period of mass murder and bombings is past, but has not yet lost its terror for Tibetans living in Tibet. Since the end of the Cultural Revolution, the Chinese occupying forces have conducted a policy of surveillance, of enforcing the introduction of Chinese customs and of tourism. Two million Tibetans now live in the Autonomous Region of Tibet. In order to diminish its geographical extent, the country was divided in 1965. Only the western third was declared an autonomous Tibetan region. Other parts of former eastern and northern Tibet now belong to the Chinese provinces of Qinghai, Sichuan, Yunnan and Gansu.

In the past few years China has invested a good deal of money in the Autonomous Region of Tibet. Roads and schools were built, and buildings and monuments of cultural and historical value were reconstructed, including the three world-famous monuments of the capital Lhasa: the Dalai Lama's winter palace, the Potala; the summer palace Norbulingka; and the Tibetan Buddhist national shrine, the Jokhang temple, as well as a few important yellow-cap monastery sites nearby. However, the reason for the renovation of these buildings was exclusively to promote tourism in the country, and legitimize Chinese rule of 'the roof of the world'. At the same time an aggressive policy of

Tibetan prayer wheels – symbols of Buddhism.

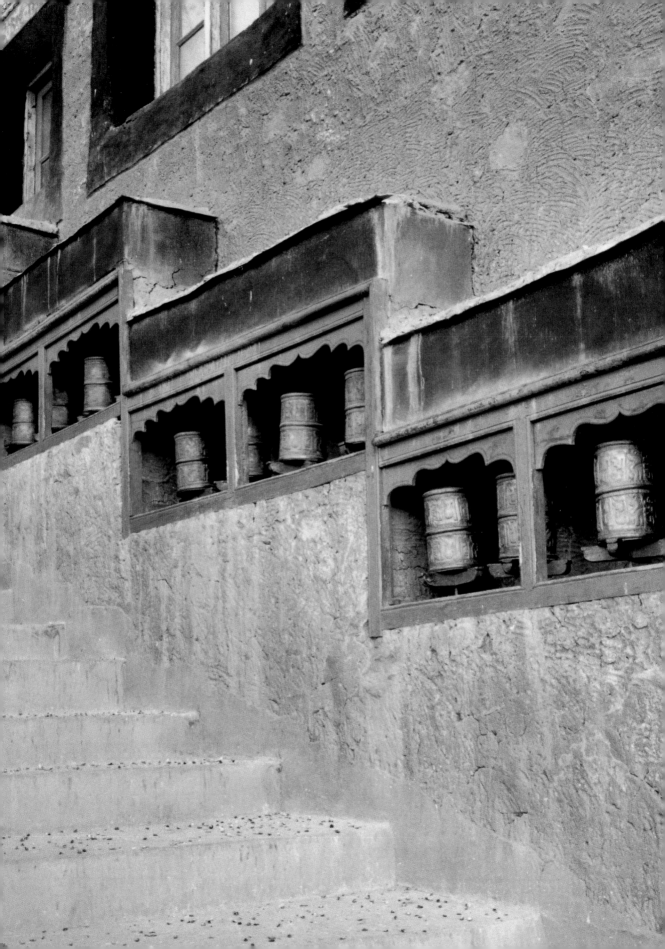

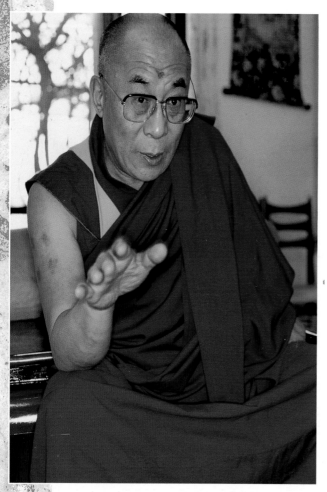

Photos of the Dalai Lama are forbidden in Tibet.

Chinese authorities have drawn up a plan called 'Lhasa 2000' which is meant to turn the capital of Tibet into a modern socialist town. Members of the Tibetan minority risk their lives if they communicate too openly with foreigners. Arrest, forced labour and torture are the order of the day. Amnesty International registered 650 political prisoners in 1995, most of whom were monks and nuns.

The official language in the Autonomous Region of Tibet is Chinese. Tibetan is only an optional extra in schools; and the children are taught that Tibet has always been part of China. While the Chinese inhabitants have remunerated work, most Tibetans are unemployed. Owing to language problems they have very few educational or work opportunities.

In the monasteries that are open to tourists, a fixed number of monks are state-subsidized, but this is mainly to provide a bit of local colour and folklore to entertain the annual influx of 80,000 tourists with their foreign currency. A few other monasteries in geographically uninviting areas have been allowed to rebuild using funds raised locally by the believers themselves (permission is required for building religious sites). Monks in these monasteries are dependent on the support of the local population, and have to provide their own food and other necessities.

Tibetan medicine has also been taken over by the Chinese. In the square in front of the Jokhang temple there is still a 'Mentsikhang', but Tibetan training and medical practice take place alongside

Chinese settlement was taking place. Around 300,000 Chinese, including 65,000 members of the police and armed forces, were tempted into the high plateau of central Tibet with high salaries and low-cost loans. In some regions, Tibetans have become a minority in their own country. Lhasa has about 200,000 inhabitants, of whom only a third or so are Tibetans. The only Tibetan houses left are around the Barkhor, a square in the old town. The

Chinese methods, such as acupuncture, and modern Western medicine, for which there is a department equipped with Western medical instruments. In the research department, Tibetan medical texts and plant-lore are studied; and on the upper floor there is a kind of library and museum for Tibetan medicine, where a few medical *thangkas* and Medicine Buddhas are on show.

In an outlying area of Lhasa stands the hospital, providing Western surgery and mainly Tibetan medical treatment. Close to the hospital is the 'College for Traditional Tibetan Medicine', but apparently the Chinese control admission to study there. It is certain that Buddhist philosophies and rituals play only a marginal role in this training. But just as before, plant-lore is on the curriculum, as well as the traditional gathering of herbs in the mountains by pupils and teachers. Linked to this college is a small factory for producing Tibetan herb pills. One department even manufactures the famous jewel or precious pills according to ancient formulae. Apparently these are much sought-after by Chinese officials in far-off Beijing. In the southern outskirts of the town, finally, there is a medicinal herb-processing factory, with large-scale production of both Western and Tibetan preparations, but there is no sign at all here of the spirit of ancient Tibetan medicine.

Monks are only just tolerated in Tibet. Many flee to India and on arrival in Dharamsala they are welcomed by an audience with the Dalai Lama.

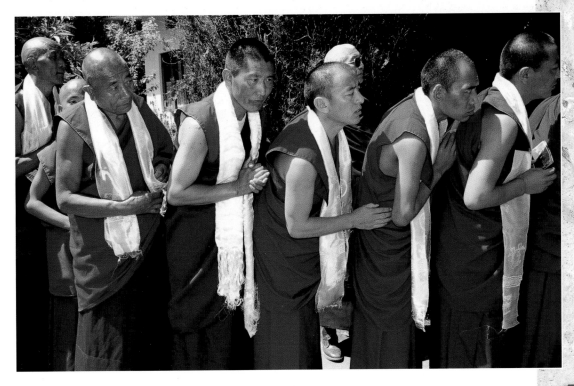

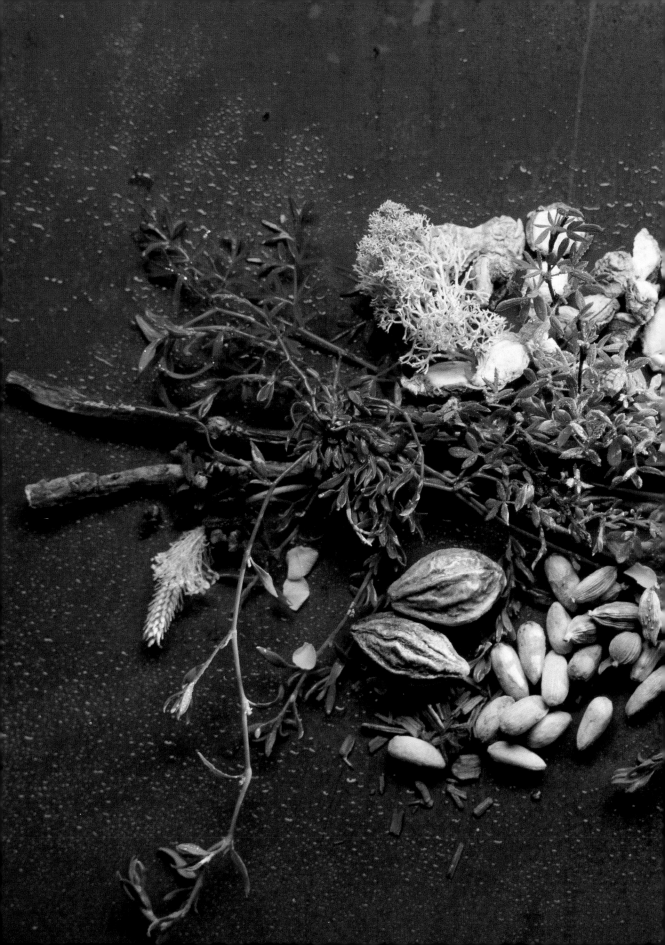

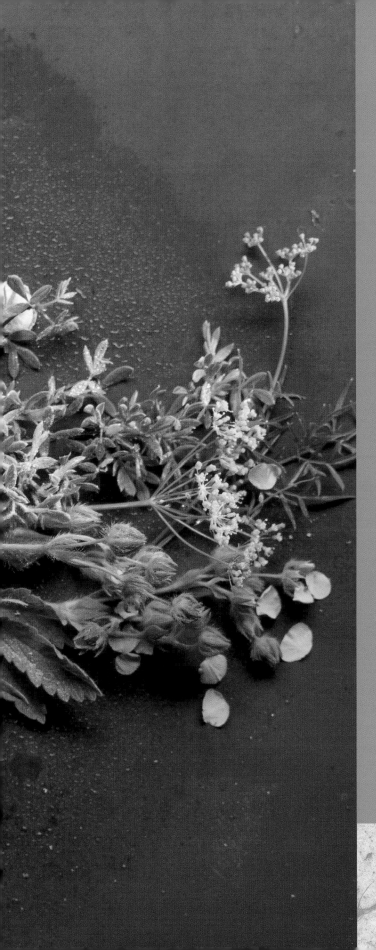

Tibetan Medicine in Europe

Chapter 5

Tibetan Doctors in the West

It is not easy to obtain medical treatments based on Tibetan practice in Europe or the USA. There are a few doctors with private clinics but so far only one, Dr Tamdin Sither Bradley, practises in the UK (for contact details, *see page 155*). Many people would be interested in training in Tibetan medicine but this is not possible in the West because the *Four Tantras* have not been completely translated. To qualify as a Tibetan physician, it is necessary to study the *Four Tantras* for a minimum of seven years, the last two of which are spent working at a branch of the Tibetan Medical and Astrological Institute in India.

However, there are a number of European groups and associations that promote Tibetan medicine. These organizations (*addresses on pages 155-6*) regularly invite well-known Tibetan doctors to give lectures or patient consultations. They also arrange training seminars for lay people and medical professionals with an interest in Tibetan medicine and diet. Contact these centres to join a waiting list for a consultation with a Tibetan doctor or to attend a lecture or conference.

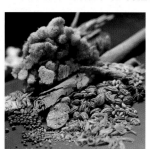

In 1998 an International Congress of Tibetan Medicine was held in Washington DC and attended by over 200 delegates: Tibetan doctors and lamas, Western doctors, scientists and psychologists. It was opened by His Holiness the Dalai Lama and considered such a success that further International Congresses are planned.

A consultation with a Tibetan doctor usually includes a pulse diagnosis and subsequent medical advice relating to diet and lifestyle based on energy type. If herbal pills or teas are recommended, these can be obtained by mail order, and they will take between two and four weeks to arrive. In Dharamsala people view mail order difficulties with Asiatic calm and composure. If anyone wants Tibetan remedies, they will find a way of obtaining them.

Padma 28

The Dalai Lama's wish to unite Tibetan medicine with Western scientific methods is already being realized in Switzerland. Padma 28, a Tibetan remedy that has been tested widely in the West, is produced just outside Zurich. Although this remedy has been on sale for over 20 years, it is only now receiving wider attention as a result of the recent surge of interest in Buddhism. Clinical trials have shown Padma 28 to be effective against arterial diseases caused by hardening of the arteries in the legs. This includes all circulatory problems, with symptoms such as tingling sensations, pins and needles or calf cramps. Professor Manuel Bicho, director of the genetics laboratory of the Lisbon medical faculty, admitted in a symposium that 'natural

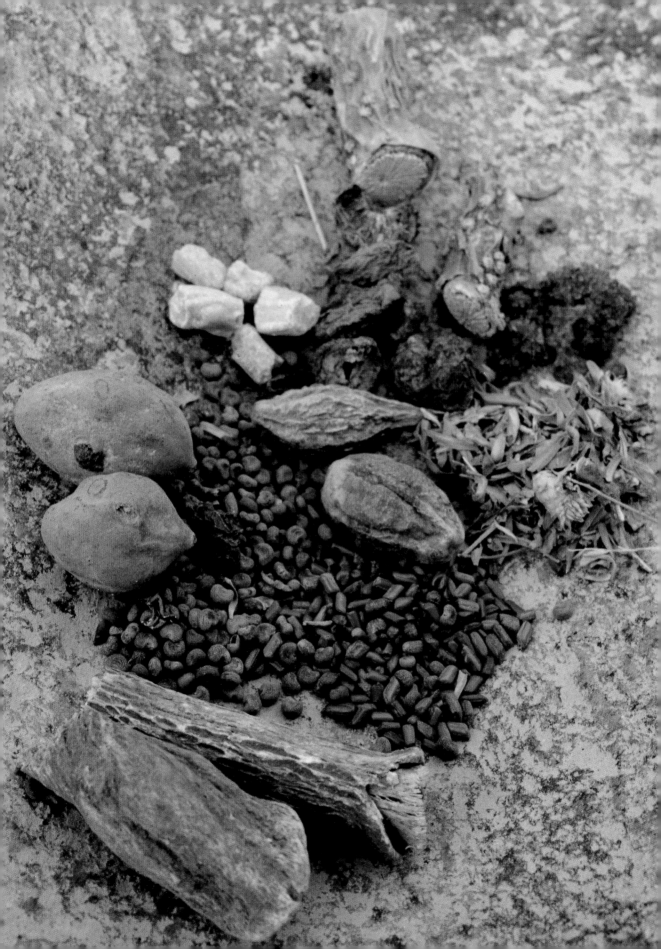

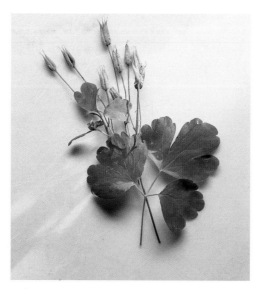

Aquilegia vulgaris or columbine – one of 20 plant ingredients in Padma 28.

herbal medicine compounds such as Padma 28, with a variety of chemical structures and biochemical and physical effects, offer a new route in prevention of the complex disease arteriosclerosis. Researchers at London's Middlesex Hospital have verified the effectiveness of Padma 28 against vascular disease and they also believe it could be very helpful in treating hepatitis B and C.

There is also evidence that, when taken regularly, Padma 28 helps to prevent hardening of the arteries. It is worth taking it as a preventative measure if risk factors such as genetic disposition, raised cholesterol levels or smoking mean there is a likelihood of such disease appearing. (According to Tibetan medicine, healthy people should not take preventative medicines, but should maintain their health through diet and lifestyle.)

Trials are underway in which Padma 28 is being used to combat coronary heart disease, chronic hepatitis B, juvenile chronic polyarthritis, and to help children with chronic respiratory infections. However, these are so far only pilot studies, so people who suffer from any of these illnesses ought not to use Padma 28 as their sole medicine, but only as a remedy to complement other therapies.

Padma 28 is a classical Tibetan compound, officially acknowledged as such by the Dalai Lama's former personal physician Yeshi Donden. 'Padma' means 'lotus flower', and the number 28 relates to a medical family's collection of remedies in which this formula was the 28th. It contains 20 different plant ingredients, including myrobalans, ribwort, valerian, marigold, columbine, icelandic moss, knotgrass, nim tree fruits, and also camphor and calcium sulphate. None of these substances alone are likely to have a specific effect but, like all Tibetan herbal remedies, Padma 28 is based on synergy: it is the combination that makes this medicine so effective.

The formula originated in Tibet but it spread to Siberia through Mongolia, whose inhabitants had strong cultural links to Tibetan Buddhism. In the middle of the 19th century the famous lama-doctor Sultim Badma, later called Alexander Badmajeff, emigrated from Siberia to St Petersburg, bringing Tibetan medicine with him to the West. In Badmajeff's suitcase, he carried a number of ancient medical formulae from the Himalayas, including Padma 28. Alexander Badmajeff's nephew, the great

Tibetan and orthodox doctor Vladimir Badmajeff who died in 1960, finally brought this herbal remedy to Poland. In the 1960s Vladimir Badmajeff's son Peter met the Swiss pharmaceuticals trader Karl Lutz, who had already spent nine years studying Tibetan medicine. Karl Lutz founded Padma Ltd in 1969, in Zollikon close to Lake Zurich, and together with Peter Badmajeff began producing Tibetan pills. So far this company is the only Western firm that manufactures Tibetan remedies.

In the UK, you will find Padma 28 in many health food shops and chemists, and the company now has a branch in Stockport, Cheshire (*see page 155 for the address*).

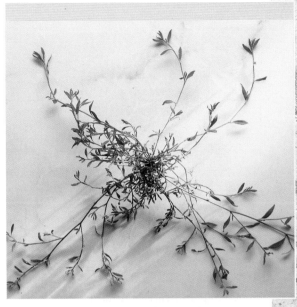

Some of the plants used in Padma 28 also grow wild in this country – such as knotgrass.

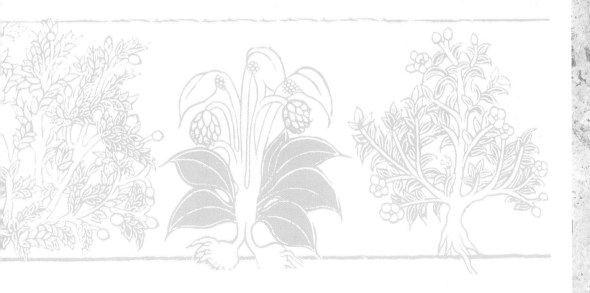

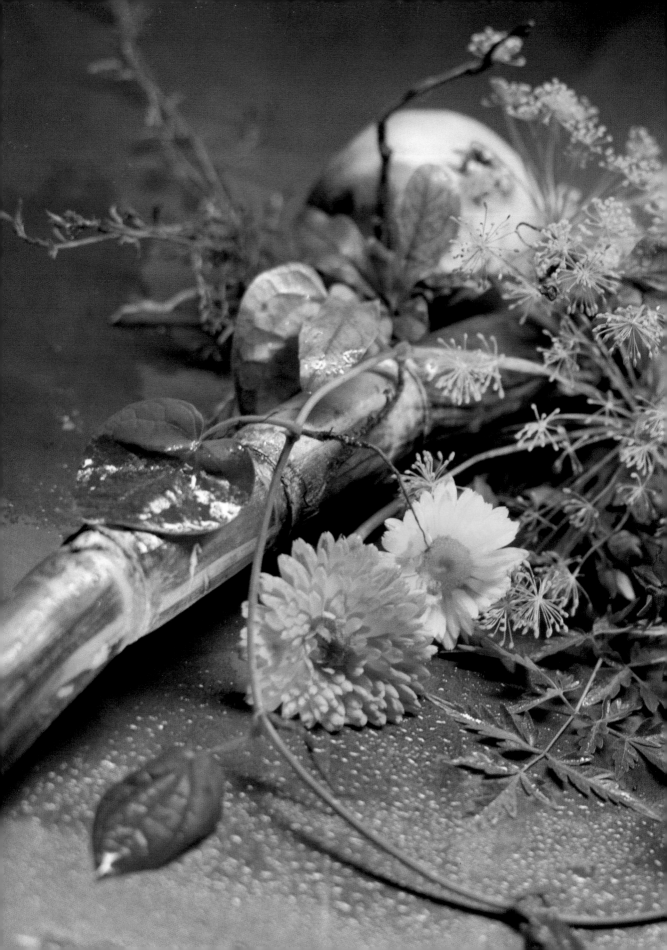

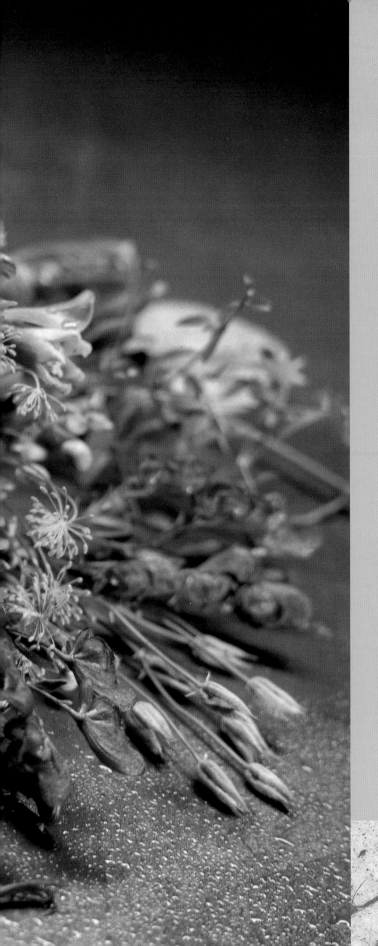

Appendices

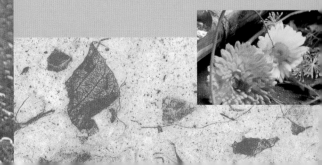

GLOSSARY

Active force
'Nuspa' in Tibetan. In some books this is referred to as 'potency'. It means the capacity of a plant, animal or mineral substance to counteract illness. Eight active forces are distinguished: heavy, oily, cool, dull, light, rough, hot and sharp.

Badkan
One of the three bodily energies, roughly translated as 'phlegm'. Relates to all bodily fluids and symbolizes everything of a heavy nature. *Badkan* illnesses are often chronic, and affect the respiratory and lymph systems among other things. At a mind-spirit level they express themselves as mental lethargy or dullness.

Blue Beryl
Also called 'Aquamarine'. A commentary on the *rGyudbzhi* written by Sangye Gyamtso in the 17th century.

Bodily energies – *see nyespa*

Formula
A prescribed medicine consisting of at least three and as many as a hundred or more individual substances.

Indigenous
A botanical concept referring to a plant's original geographical area of distribution.

Mkhrispa
One of the three bodily energies, which can be roughly translated as 'bile', but which only has a distant relationship to the bodily fluid of the same name. It symbolizes all bodily processes linked to metabolism and combustion. *Mkhrispa* disorders manifest, among other things, as infections and inflammations; and at a mind-spirit level as aggression or fanaticism.

Nyespa
The concept of the three bodily energies *rlung*, *mkhrispa* and *badkan*, the harmonization of which is the aim of Tibetan medicine. Other terms for this are the three fluids, life essences or energy principles. The Tibetan teaching of the three energies derives from the Ayurvedic teaching of the three *doshas* (juices). The literal translation of *nyespa*, 'harm-causer', refers to the three mind poisons corresponding to the energies. These are greed (*rlung*), hatred (*mkhrispa*) and blindness (*badkan*), which are thought to be the cause of all physical and emotional or mental suffering.

rGyudbzhi
A fundamental text book on Tibetan medicine, still pertinent in the 21st century. It was probably written in the 12th century by Yuthog Gonpo. It has four parts, the *Four Tantras*, of which only two have so far been translated into a Western language. Medical students still learn the *rGyudbzhi* by heart.

rlung
The most important of the three bodily energies, also called 'wind energy'. Stands for the life-sustaining principle and for all that moves in the body. *Rlung* disorders often manifest as stress symptoms, as muscular tensions of the back or as diseases of the nervous system.

Taste, taste sphere

Ro in Tibetan. Tibetan medicine divides all medicinal plants and foods into the following six taste spheres: sweet, sour, salty, bitter, sharp and astringent. See also *zurjes*.

Thangka

Translated, this means 'picture' or 'painting', and refers to a scroll picture framed in silk. The medicine *thangkas* are 79 scroll pictures that were painted in the 17th century to illustrate the whole of Tibetan medical lore.

Tsa

The subtle energy in the meridians.

Yontan

Tibetan for 'qualities'. According to Tibetan categorization, remedies and foods are divided into 17 different qualities, including dry, heavy, light, oily, sharp and rough.

Zurjes

Tibetan for 'post-digestive taste', or 'taste after digestion'. Each medicinal herb has both a taste and a taste after digestion, which are not always the same. There are three *zurjes*: sweet, sour, bitter. For instance, some plants of salty taste have a sweet 'post-digestive' taste.

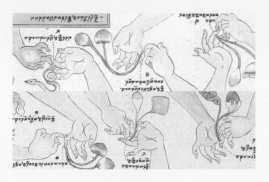

USEFUL ADDRESSES
Tibetan medicine in Europe

UK:

For a Tibetan doctor practising in the UK, contact:
Dr Tamdin S. Bradley
17 Frating Crescent
Woodford Green
Essex IG8 0DW
Tel/fax: 020 8504 1026
email: drtamdin@freeuk.com

For general information on Tibet, including details of doctors visiting from India, contact:
Tibet Foundation
10 Bloomsbury Way
London WC1A 2SH
Tel: 020 7405 5284

You can obtain the incense sticks Agar 31 and Golar 25 from:
The Kailash Centre of Oriental Medicine
7 Newcourt Street
London NW8 7AA
Tel: 020 7722 3939
Fax: 020 7722 7878
The centre also arranges yoga groups. It is necessary to attend an induction course before joining these closed groups.

Padma 28 can be obtained by mail order from:
Padma 28 (UK) Ltd
Hazel Grove
Stockport
Cheshire SK7 5BW
Tel: 0161 483 4662

You will also find Padma teas in selected health food shops and chemists in the UK.

Switzerland

Dr Tendhon Amipa-Desam
Gemeinschaftspraxis Dres. Gunsch & Kählin
Rosengasse 9
CH-8332 Russikon
Swizerland
Tel: 00 41 195 42111
Tel and fax for private clients:
00 41 186 56415

Dr Kalsang Shak
Arbachstrasse 56
CH-6340 Baar
Switzerland
Tel/fax: 00 41 417 608135
Tibetan health counselling, and seminars on Tibetan medicine and Tibetan Buddhism.

Padma AG
Dammstrasse 29
CH-8702 Zollikon
Switzerland
Tel: 00 41 1391 9555
Fax: 00 41 1391 9818
For herbal remedies.

Tibet Institut Rikon
Sekretariat, Wildbergstrasse
CH-8486 Rikon
Switzerland
Tel: 00 41 5238 1729
For information on Tibetan Buddhism.

For information on the GYU.LAM.DOL method, contact:
Antonia Yeshe Dechen Strub-Tusch
Seestrasse 2

CH-8330 Pfäffikon
Switzerland
Tel: 00 41 1951 1601
Fax: 00 41 1955 1702

Italy

Dr Pasang Yonten Arya
Via Carnavali Antonio 111
I- 20158 Milan
Italy
Tel: 00 39 2659 21 93
Fax: 00 39 23761 863

Yuthok, Institute for Tibetan Medicine
Via Francanzano 11
I- 80127 Napoli
Italy
Tel/fax: 00 39 815 789946

Holland

NSTG/TMAI
Prinsengracht 200
Amsterdam
1016 MD Holland
Tel: 00 31 20 404 4747
Fax: 00 31 20 624 2810

In the clinic linked to this institute, a Tibetan doctor from the Dharamsala Medical and Astrological Institute is always available. There is also a dispensary where Tibetan herb remedies and precious pills can be obtained on prescription.

Austria

Florian Lauda
Postgasse 11
A-1010 Vienna
Austria
Tel: 00 43 151 226 86

Germany

Tibetisches Zentrum e.v
Hermann-Balk-Strasse 106
D-22147 Hamburg
Germany
Tel: 00 49 40 644 3585
Fax: 00 49 40 644 3515

Aryatara Institut
Barerstrasse 70/Rgb.
D-80799 Munich
Germany
Tel: 00 49 8927 81 7227
Fax: 00 49 8927 81 7226

For information and training courses on Kum
Nye yoga, contact:
Matthias Steurich
Im Oberdorf 1
D-79292 Pfaffenweiler
Germany
Tel and fax: 00 49 7664 609 66
He also produces books and exercise videos.

TIBETAN MEDICINE
IN ASIA

India

**The Medical and Astrological Institute
(Men-Tsee-Khang) in Dharamsala**
Gangchen Kyishong
Dharamsala 176215
District Kangra (H.P.)
Tel: 00 91 1892 231 13 or 226 18
Fax: 0091 1892 241 16
email: tmai@dsala.tibet.net

On request the Institute can supply the
addresses of its 38 branches in India and 2
branches in Nepal.

In Delhi:
Tibetan Medical Institute
13, Jaipur Estate Nizamuddin
East New Delhi 110013
India
Tel: 00 91 11 469 85 03 (clinic)
00 91 11 463 50 99 (office)
At this, the largest branch of the Medical and
Astrological Institute, you can order Sorig
products, such as incense sticks, Sorig Tea
and ointment.

Treatment via letter:
The Dharamsala Medical and Astrological
Institute offers 'consultations by letter' to
patients abroad. For this you need to
describe the history of your illness in detail,
in English. The letter will be presented to
one of the Dalai Lama's three personal
physicians, Dr Tenzin Choedrak, Dr Lobsang
Wangyal or Dr Kunga Gyurme. The medicine
prescribed by one of these doctors will be
sent to the required address on receipt of
payment.

Dr Tenzin Choedrak
The personal physician of His Holiness the
14th Dalai Lama took part in a documentary
film by Franz Reichle on Tibetan medicine,
entitled *Das Wissen vom Heilen* ('Knowledge
of healing'). A video can be obtained from:
Naturheilverein Zell u.A. e.V
Postfach
D-73119 Zell u.A.
Germany

BIBLIOGRAPHY

Arya, Dr Pasaang Yonten and Gyatso, Dr Yonten, *Dictionary of Tibetan Materia Medica*, Motilal Banarsidass, 1998

Burang, Theodore, *The Tibetan Art of Healing*, London 1974

Clifford, Terry, *Tibetan Buddhist Medicine and Psychiatry,* Samuel Weiser, 1984

Cornu, Philippe, *Tibetan Astrology*, Shambhala Publications, 1997

Dalai Lama, *The Art of Happiness*, Hodder & Stoughton, 1998
– *MindScience*, with Dr Herbert Benson et al., Wisdom Publications, 1991

Donden, Dr Yeshi, *Health Through Balance,* Snow Lion Publications, 1986 – *The Ambrosia Heart Tantra*, Vol. 1, annotated by Yeshi Donden, Library of Tibetan Works and Archives, Dharamsala, 1977

Finkh, Elisabeth, *Studies in Tibetan Medicine*, 1978

Meyer, Fernand, *Tibetan Medical Paintings*, Serindia Publications, 1992

Norbu, Dawa, *An Introduction to Tibetan Medicine*, Tibetan Review Publications, Delhi, 1976

Rinpoche, Dr Akong Tulke, *Taming the Tiger*, Rider Books, 1992

Rinpoche, Sogyal, *Tibetan Book of Living and Dying*, Rider Books, 1992

Tsarong, Tsewang J, *Tibetan Medical Plants*, Tibetan Medical Publications, 1994

Source literature for the chapter on plants

Clark, Barry (trans.): *Rgyud bzi – The Quintessence Tantras of Tibetan Medicine*, Snow Lion Publications, Ithaca/New York 1988

Dash, Vaidya: *Bhagwan: Materia Medica of Tibetan Medicine*, Sri Satguru Publications, Delhi 1994

Dash, Vaidya: *Bhagwan: Materia Medica of Indo-Tibetan Medicine*, Classics India Publications, Delhi 1989

Franke, Wolfgang: *Nutzpflanzenkunde, Thieme*, Stuttgart/New York 1981

Haupt, Paul: *Klassische tibetische Medizin*, Bern/Stuttgart/Vienna 1996

List, Ph.; Hörhammer, L: *Hagers Handbuch der pharmazeutischen Praxis*, Springer, Berlin/Heidelberg 1992

Orient Longmann, P.K.Warrier, V.P.K. Nambiar, C. Ramankutty (eds.): *Indian Medicinal Plants, Ltd.*, Chennai 1996

SMan-sTsis, vol. 1, no. 1, TMAI, Dharamsala 1995

Tsarong, Tsewang J.: *Tibetan Medicinal Plants*, Tibetan Medical Publications, Kalimpong 1994

Tsarong, Tsewang J.: *Handbook of Traditional Tibetan Drugs*, Tibetan Medical Publications, Kalimpong 1986

Zander, Robert; Encke, Fritz; Buchheim, Günther; Seybold, Siegmund (eds.): *Handwörterbuch der Pflanzennamen, Ulmer*, Stuttgart 1994